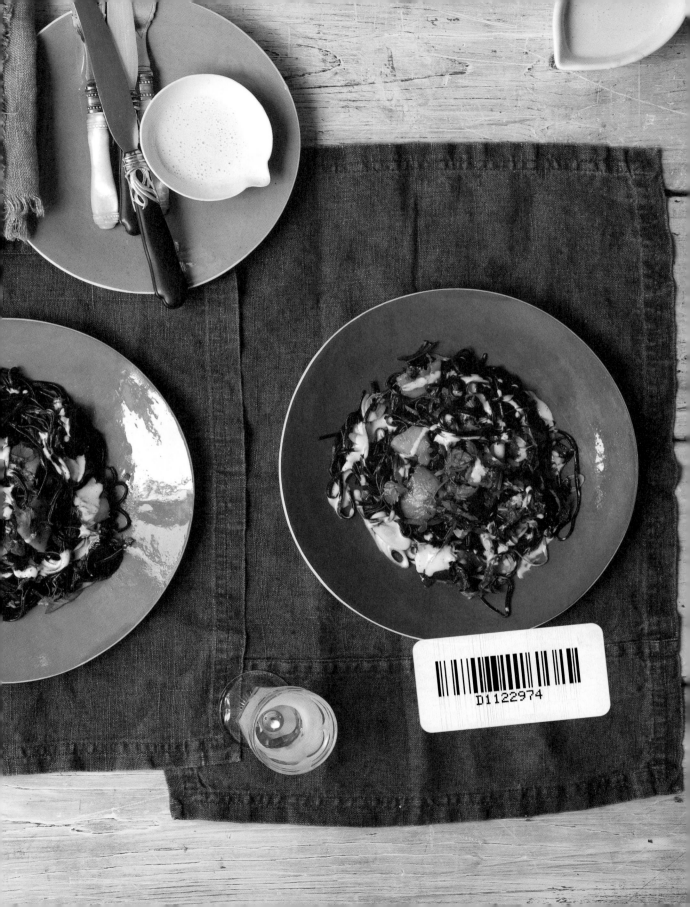

D1122974

HONESTLY
HEALTHY
FOR LIFE

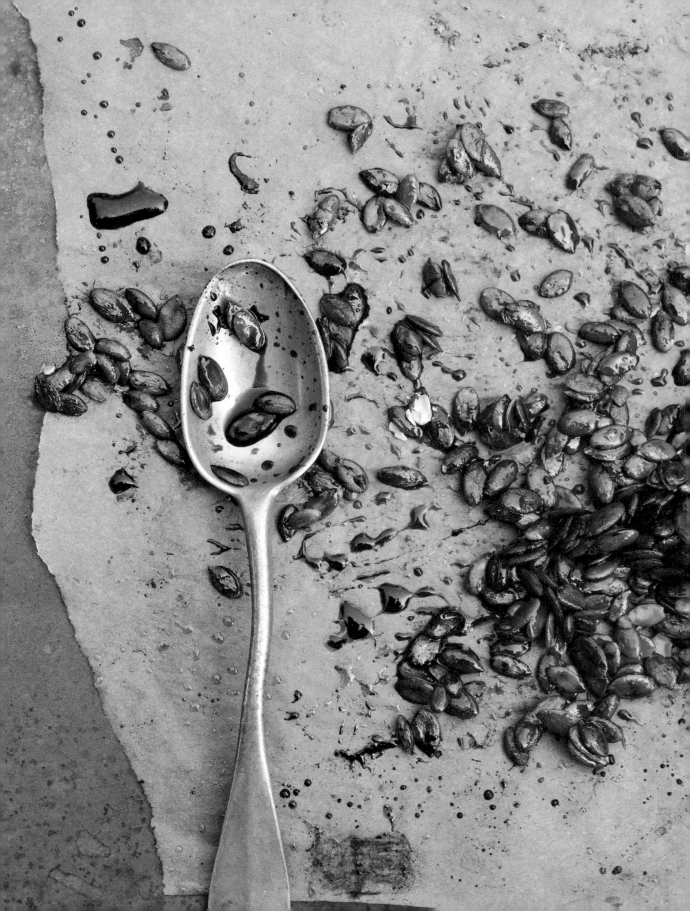

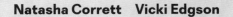

Natasha Corrett   Vicki Edgson

HONESTLY HEALTHY FOR LIFE

Eating the Alkaline Way Every Day

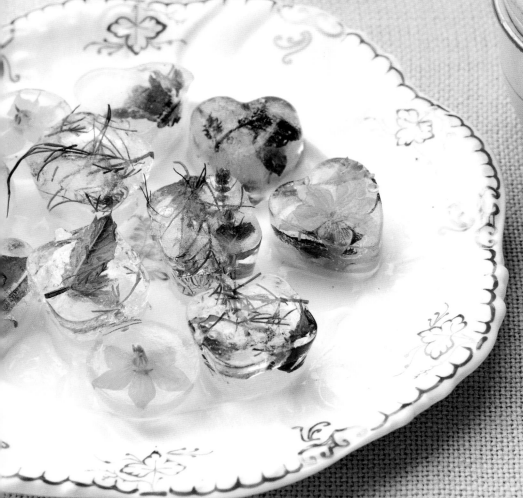

Photography by Lisa Linder

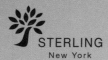

STERLING
New York

For information about custom editions, special sales, and premium and corporate purchases, please contact Sterling Special Sales at 800-805-5489 or specialsales@sterlingpublishing.com.

Manufactured in China

10 9 8 7 6 5 4 3 2 1

www.sterlingpublishing.com

Key to symbols for alkaline ratings

 Really really alkaline recipe

 Really alkaline recipe

 Alkaline recipe

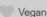 Vegan

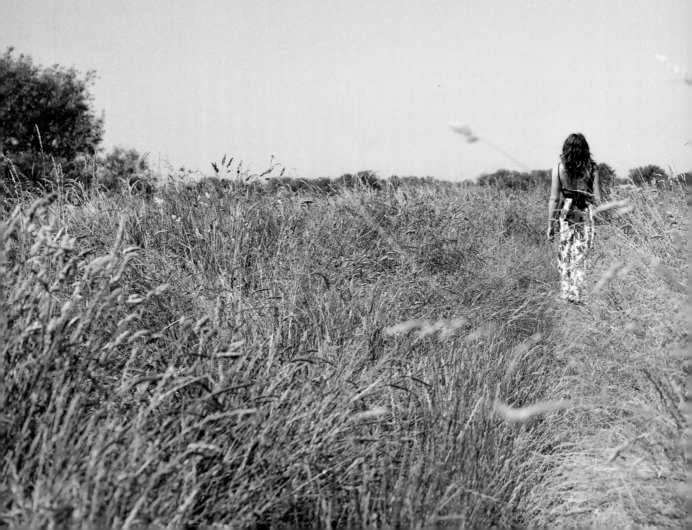

From Tash
To the most inspirational woman in my life—my amazing grandmother, Stephanie, who is a true friend and a sensational support.

From Vix
To all my thousands of clients, who have inspired me with their learning and findings just as much as my knowledge of nutrition. We are on this journey together.

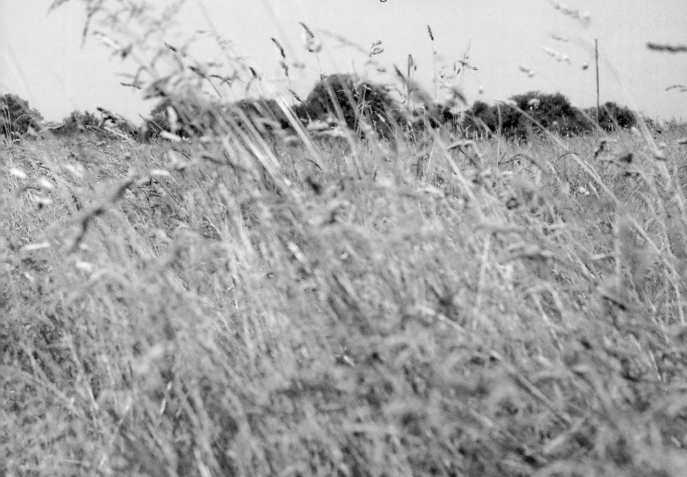

INTRODUCTION

Since the first Honestly Healthy book—*Eating the Alkaline Way*—was published in 2012, eating alkaline has gained huge momentum as an ideal way to eat for energy, health, and well-being using delicious organic ingredients, and has been embraced by the media as a popular way to manage what you eat.

We were totally delighted—and, it has to be said, utterly surprised—by the huge success of the first book along with the thousands of inquiries we had about the principles behind alkaline eating and a desire for more recipes. So, we turned our attention and energies to answer the demand. The result? This book—*Honestly Healthy For Life*—embraces how the alkaline way of eating can fit into your everyday life. Whether it's lazy weekends and breakfast in bed, snacks to take while traveling with work, weekday suppers, delicious cakes and treats, crowd-pleasing dishes for celebratory meals, or great nights in with friends, you'll find we have inspirational and accessible recipes to fit any occasion or celebration.

In its simplest form, eating alkaline means that you adopt a predominantly vegetarian approach to food. To ensure you eat the best combinations of nutrients, we recommend a variety of vegetables along with legumes, nuts, and seeds, sprouted and living foods from the land and sea (which supply the body-building and repairing proteins). In this book, we clearly explain what is an alkaline food (and what's an acid-forming food) as well as present an at-a-glance chart of the alkaline ratings of commonly eaten foods (see pages 14–15).

Soon after the publication of the first book, Tash's Fridge Fill service (which delivers Honestly Healthy daily meals to your door) started to grow rapidly as a result of those clients, friends, and general inquiries that came from the success of the book. Soon Tash was to be found bound to her kitchen in order to supply the ever-growing demand, but we were delighted that so many people were responding so positively to the information and recipes in the book. Fridge Fill has now become a full-time business in its own right, with Tash steering weekly menus that are delivered all over the UK. It's simply wonderful for us to see the message of the positive benefits of alkaline eating reaching an ever-wider audience.

As readers of the first book will attest, eating nutritious meals doesn't mean depriving yourself of anything. Homemade treats are thankfully never off the menu and are far better—taste-wise and nutrient-wise—as our recipes use natural sweeteners (fruits and spices or naturally sourced sugars, for instance), rather than those commercially produced items that are laden with refined sugars (among the most acid-forming of all foods). And if you feel that you can't live without animal protein of some kind, you will find an abundance of recipes that can have a small amount added; that said, we like to encourage all of our readers to try taking the vegetarian route for just three weeks to see how much better they feel.

Gatherings of friends and family are a big part of our lives, so cooking dishes that suit everyone is high up on our agenda. Tash has created lots of recipes that are easy to scale up for birthday celebrations or parties in the garden that cater to all tastes and all ages. Let's face it, who's ever too old for a gingerbread man, fruit ice pop, or a slice of birthday cake? It's great to know that all members of a family can eat the alkaline way; our recipes supply all the vital nutrients for growing children and adults of all ages. And why would you eat ready-made sandwiches or pasta dinners when you could be tucking into Mini Sushi Rolls, Roasted Tomato and Spinach Tart, or Raw Green Curry with Zucchini "Noodles"? When eating the Honestly Healthy way, no one goes hungry since you're fully nourished by nature's nutrient-dense foods.

As more research is highlighting the potentially damaging and life-suppressing effects of mass-produced food, much of which we would be hard-pressed to find in nature, we are now encouraging all our readers (new as well as devoted), to get back into the kitchen, to

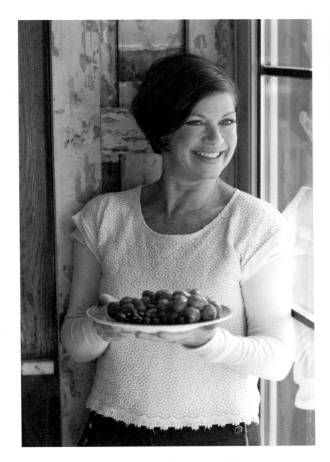

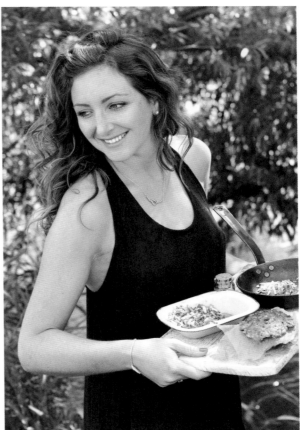

select their own raw ingredients, and be aware of what they are putting into their mouths. It is no coincidence that obesity and diabetes are on the rise, skin problems are everywhere, chaotic hormone-related diseases are now pandemic, and cancers affect more than one in three adults and children worldwide. We have to ask the obvious question—why is this happening in a world where medical research has never been as advanced as it is now? One of those answers must be "because of the foods we are eating."

But sourcing organic and wholesome ingredients doesn't have to mean sky-high shopping bills. Share in the joys of nature by growing your own ingredients—herbs and small vegetables—whether in boxes on windowsills or in gardens. The taste of home-grown produce really is hard to beat. As well as supplying a regular source of ingredients, growing your own is easy and low cost; plus it offers everyone a way to connect with nature and to understand "where food comes

from." Whether weight is an issue for you or not, we know that following the alkaline eating way is simply the safest, longest-lasting method for permanent weight loss—it allows your body to find its perfect size. Alkaline eating helps your body to get what it needs from good-quality food, resulting in the right body for you, with a lower body mass index and a trimmer figure.

So, we encourage you to turn the pages of this book, salivate over the mouth-watering recipes (and please do make them, rather than just look at the beautiful pictures), and see for yourself how quickly your energy will soar, your ills will abate, and you will regain your former, younger self. We know it works because we are both living proof, and the tens of thousands of readers of the first book agree, too. So, here's to *Honestly Healthy for Life*!

Tash x Vicki

Tash and Vicki

KNOW YOUR ACID FROM YOUR ALKALINE

The last time you might have come across the term "pH" was during a school chemistry class and it's probably not something you've ever thought of with respect to food. But getting to grips with the basics of acid and alkaline in terms of food is simple—we'll show you how—and it helps to explain why alkaline eating benefits your body.

Don't rely on a food's taste

You may think you can tell which foods are acid and which are alkaline by how they taste, but you'd be wrong. There are many foods that taste neutral, such as yogurt, that when digested become acidic in the digestive system. And, lemon or lime for instance, might taste acidic, but when digested these become alkaline.

When you eat food, it is digested by various enzymes secreted in the mouth, stomach, and eventually small intestines. The digested form of a food is what we call its "ash" and it is different from the original food. The ash of a food is the fully digested version that is broken down into a liquid state, ready for absorption into the bloodstream, for transport around the body so it's available to all body cells wherever they are.

Typically, the ash of foods that taste tart on the tongue, such as citrus fruits, tomatoes, pickled vegetables (like ginger or Japanese umeboshi plums), actually become alkaline, with the added benefit of improving your digestive function as a result. Whereas some foods, such as meat, dairy produce, and refined cereals, produce an acidic ash and become acid-forming in the body. This transformation during the digestive process is the most important concept to grasp, as it is not the taste that counts, but rather the effect it has on the digestive system as a whole.

When your body is bombarded with acid-forming foods, it has to rely on supplies within your body to recalibrate your blood pH so that it stays within its strict limits, which can mean leaching minerals out of your bone tissue or putting extra work on your kidneys and liver.

What is pH?
The values of pH are measured from 0 to 14: those values from 0 to 6.9 are acidic; those values from 7.1 to 14 are alkaline; while 7 is said to be neutral.

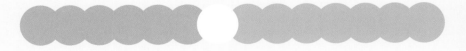

For your body to work optimally, all the biochemical reactions that take place to supply you with energy, digest your food, and control your mood (to name but a few) have to take place in controlled conditions. The pH of blood sits in a narrow range of 7.35–7.45, slightly alkaline, and your body does everything it can to maintain this value.

Easy on the body

Alkaline foods are easier to digest, improving immune function in the gut as a direct result and automatically banishing indigestion, bloating, and gas. And not all vegetables and fruit are equal. Most vegetables, particularly green vegetables, are highly alkaline, while only some fruits (such as avocados and tomatoes) produce an alkaline or neutral ash when they have been digested.

As you'll see in the recipe section, there is no shortage of treats available when you eat alkaline foods. Fruits can be simmered down to produce a concentrated natural form of sugar that is alkaline, so you can get a sweet hit from this rather than snacking solely on soft fruit, such as raspberries and strawberries, that are more acidic (and, coincidentally, are two of the fruits with the highest food intolerance ratings).

To find out which commonly eaten foods are alkaline and which are acid-forming (and where they sit along the pH spectrum), refer to the simple chart on pages 14–15.

An inflammatory situation

As well as overworking your digestive system, acid-forming foods lead to inflammation and mucus production. Think of anyone you know who always has a tissue to hand for their constantly runny nose (rhinitis) or what is known as a post-nasal drip (constantly having a sense of catarrh running down the back of the throat or needing to clear the throat a lot). Inflammatory conditions range from the skin (eczema and psoriasis) through bones, muscles, and joints (arthritis and swollen joints) to the large intestine (Crohn's disease and ulcerative colitis). Such conditions can be debilitating, life-changing, and, needless to say, intensely painful.

Abundant research has indicated that most heart disease also starts with inflammation, and that controlling the inflammation is the key to lowering the risk of heart attack and stroke. Most medical doctors prescribe synthetic anti-inflammatory medications, but wouldn't it be superb if they were taught about nature's own versions, such as nuts and seeds, and their oils (think olive, sunflower, avocado, and walnut oils)?

The chia seed, which originated as a nutrition source in South America during the times of the Incas, has now been evaluated as being the highest source of vegetarian omega-3 essential fatty acids—the primary anti-inflammatory food. (See page 22 for more on vegetarian sources of omega-3 fats and page 63 for a delicious breakfast recipe with this versatile ingredient.)

It's all about balance

As you'll read in later chapters, what we recommend at Honestly Healthy is eating predominantly alkaline foods (we recommend 70% alkaline:30% acid-forming foods), not 100% alkaline foods. When you eat foods based on the 70:30 ratio, you'll feel more satisfied on less food, as all alkaline foods tend to nourish without requiring excessive energy to digest them, thereby balancing blood sugar levels and providing you with more energy. We'll talk about how best to achieve this ratio later (see page 42).

Eating alkaline is not a simple case of calories in vs calories out, as is more usually measured in determining whether or not a food is good for you or for weight management, but rather it focuses on the nutrient density of foods and their bio-availability once digested.

When we talk of nutrient density, what we mean is the abundance of specific and combined nutrients that any one food provides, including protein, antioxidants, and essential fats. If we take avocado as a food, a calorie-counting approach makes it one to avoid as it is high in calories, but what calorie counting fails to appreciate is that it's a rich source of protein, essential fats, and antioxidant vitamins—making avocados a perfect superfood. In the alkaline approach we view this aspect of a food as much more important than calories per se. In addition, some foods, such as dark green leafy vegetables, release their nutrients more readily than others, making it easier for your body to digest and obtain what it needs.

Most alkaline foods, such as lemons, limes, celery, watercress, spinach, kale, and chard, are packed with nutrient-laden water. This mineral-rich water is more easily absorbed than plain bottled water, as the glucose molecules in each of these foods help to carry the water across the cell membrane of those organs where the hydration is most needed. This allows you to hydrate the body from food and not just from drinking water. At the other end of the scale, all animal produce is acid-forming when digested, taking far longer to break down into its component parts and requiring abundant stomach acid to complete even the first

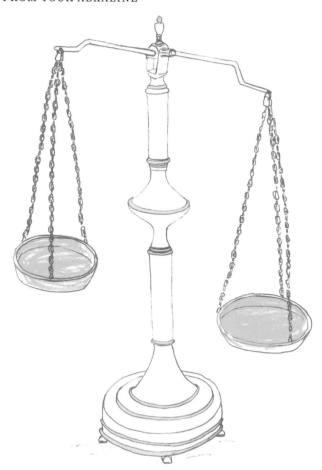

stage of digestion. This may not be troublesome to youngsters and teenagers, whose digestive systems are usually robust. However, for anyone under stress, studying under pressure, working long hours, pregnant, or elderly, the production of stomach acid may be lowered or suppressed, leading to heartburn, burping, nausea, and pain upon eating. The now all-too-familiar condition of lactose intolerance (an intolerance to cow's dairy produce, in particular) that afflicts so many adults around the world today is a perfect example of how acid-forming foods can overload and overwhelm the digestive system.

If you've ever overheard someone saying "I can't eat red meat, it sits in my system for days," well that's because it's true. Red meats, chicken, and other poultry are all acid-forming, and they can take up to four days to be broken down in the digestive tract, leading to symptoms such as constipation, headaches, skin outbreaks (a sign of toxicity in the gut), and even depression.

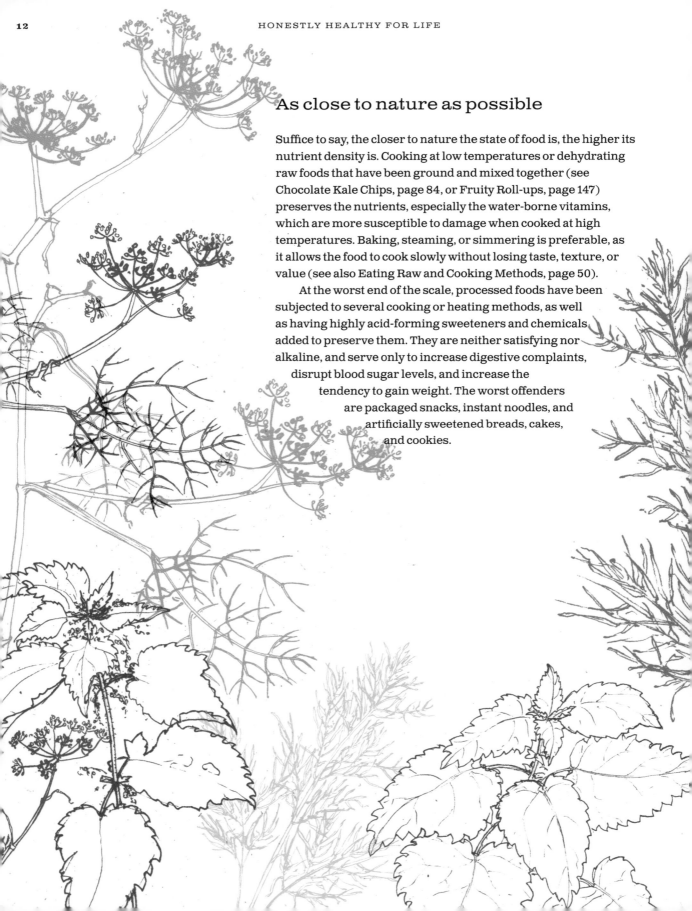

As close to nature as possible

Suffice to say, the closer to nature the state of food is, the higher its nutrient density is. Cooking at low temperatures or dehydrating raw foods that have been ground and mixed together (see Chocolate Kale Chips, page 84, or Fruity Roll-ups, page 147) preserves the nutrients, especially the water-borne vitamins, which are more susceptible to damage when cooked at high temperatures. Baking, steaming, or simmering is preferable, as it allows the food to cook slowly without losing taste, texture, or value (see also Eating Raw and Cooking Methods, page 50).

At the worst end of the scale, processed foods have been subjected to several cooking or heating methods, as well as having highly acid-forming sweeteners and chemicals added to preserve them. They are neither satisfying nor alkaline, and serve only to increase digestive complaints, disrupt blood sugar levels, and increase the tendency to gain weight. The worst offenders are packaged snacks, instant noodles, and artificially sweetened breads, cakes, and cookies.

WHAT ALTERS THE pH OF FOOD?

So, we know that the pH of a food can change from its natural state to its digested ash. What's more, states within the body can affect bodily functions, including digestion (which is inextricably linked with emotions), so it's no surprise that negative emotions, stress, upsetting natural rhythms (international travel), and micronutrient deficiency can all affect how a food is processed and absorbed.

Help your body to help itself Your body naturally produces enzymes to digest food on a constant basis, but lack of sleep, traveling internationally on a frequent basis, and negative emotions (such as anger, frustration, and depression) can profoundly affect this production, as the body places more of its energy on managing these issues than it does on digestive function itself.

Positive pick-me-ups At Honestly Healthy we advocate conscious eating, making sure you're aware of whatever you're putting in your mouth (see page 47). But for some it's all too easy to reach for food for a pick-me-up. If you "eat on an emotion"—for instance, if you are upset with someone or feel you have been let down—you are more likely to choose foods that don't nourish you, arguing that you "deserve this" to try to ameliorate the negative emotion. But we at Honestly Healthy know that the only way to comfort yourself positively is to drink or eat alkaline foods—so instead of reaching for a chocolate cookie, whiz up a great green smoothie with avocado, broccoli, and watercress (see page 64) or munch a homemade Raw Hemp Granola Bar (see page 87) and take care of yourself, rather than adding insult to injury.

Don't fall for "mindless sandwich syndrome" When you're stressed and finding it difficult to cope with situations, your body produces lots of a hormone called cortisol. Cortisol's original function is to help ready the body for "fight or flight," but as it diverts attention to muscles and away from the digestive system, it lowers the production of stomach acid, which in turn makes it more difficult to break down all types of food, especially protein. If you're too busy to eat, don't just grab and go and hope that it fills you up—eating too quickly and without concentrating on what you are eating is what we call the "mindless sandwich syndrome." Take more time and care to choose what will nourish you—wheat-based bread is highly acidic, as are most of the fillers that come in sandwiches, so opt for a Salad Wrap (see page 69), Lyra's Pesto (see page 110), or Tash's Famous Hummus (see page 211) with vegetable crudités.

Maximize micronutrients Both magnesium and vitamin C are important for buffering the kidneys from excessive acid-forming foods or acidic ashes (see page 9). So be sure to top up on magnesium-rich and vitamin C-rich foods. Magnesium is found in richest supply in dark green leafy vegetables that are highest on the alkaline spectrum. In fact, eating foods from the Really Really Alkaline and Really Alkaline lists (see pages 14–15) every day is a fast-track way to ensure that you are providing yourself with ample magnesium and abundant vitamin C. We cannot store vitamin C in the body so we have to eat vitamin C-rich foods daily to access this important antioxidant to ensure that we have ample protection from oxidative free radicals produced in the body in response to stress. Not surprisingly, vitamin C is found in richest supply in those fruits and vegetables that are the highest on the alkaline spectrum.

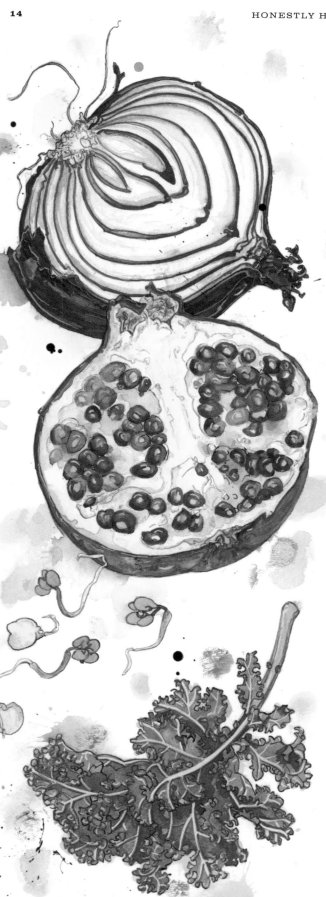

FROM ALKALINE SUPERFOODS TO DEFINITE NO-NOS

Really really alkaline	Really alkaline
Almonds	Arugula
Apple cider vinegar	Avocado
Broccoli	Basil
Celtic sea salt	Bee pollen
Chard	Beet
Cucumber	Cabbage
Endive	Celery
Fennel	Chia (also known as salba)
Grasses *wheatgrass, barley, kamut grass, etc.*	Chinese cabbage
Himalayan pink salt	Chives
Kale	Cilantro
Flat-leaf parsley	Eggplant
pH 9.5 alkaline water	Escarole
Sea vegetables *kelp, nori, wakame*	Figs
Spinach	Garlic
Sprouts *soy, alfalfa, pumpkin, sunflower, broccoli, amaranth, sesame, chia*	Ginger
	Green beans
Sprouted beans *aduki, chickpea, lentils, mung beans, split peas*	Jerusalem artichoke
	Lemon
	Lettuce
	Lima beans
	Lime
	Mustard greens
	Navy beans
	Okra
	Onion
	Peppers (all colors)
	Quinoa
	Radish
	Red onion
	Scallion
	Spring greens
	Tomato

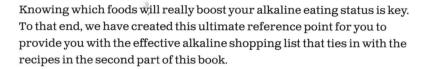
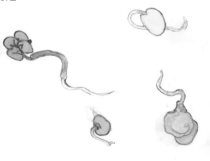

Knowing which foods will really boost your alkaline eating status is key. To that end, we have created this ultimate reference point for you to provide you with the effective alkaline shopping list that ties in with the recipes in the second part of this book.

Alkaline	Quite alkaline	Less alkaline	Acidic
Almond milk	Black beans	Apple	Alcohol
Artichoke	Brazil nut	Apricot	Beef
Asparagus	Brown rice	Banana	Black tea
Avocado oil	Buckwheat flour *in breads and pasta or noodles*	Blackberry	Chicken and other poultry
Brussels sprouts	Cantaloupe	Blueberry	Cocoa
Buckwheat	Caught wild fish	Canned sweetcorn	Coffee
Carrot	Couscous	Chickpeas	Corn syrup
Cashew nuts	Fresh date	Chilis	Dairy produce *milk, cheese, yogurt*
Cauliflower	Grapeseed oil	Cranberry	Dried fruit
Chestnuts	Greengage	Fresh, natural juice *such as mango, peach, and apricot*	Eggs
Coconut flesh, milk, and water	Hazelnuts	Goat's cheese	Farmed fish
Coconut oil	Millet	Grapes	Gelatin
Fava beans	Mushrooms	Guava	Honey
Flax oil or Udo's oil *mixed vegetable-sourced omega 3/6 oil as supplement*	Nectarine	Kidney beans	Jam
Goat's milk	Oats	Kiwi	Ketchup
Grapefruit	Pecans	Mango	Lamb
Herbs and spices *thyme, mint, ginger, cumin, etc.*	Pear	Mangosteen	Miso (and all other fermented foods)
Leeks	Pearl barley	Mayonnaise	Pork
Lentils	Pine nuts	Ocean fish	Ready-made mustard
New potatoes	Pistachios	Orange	Rice syrup
Olive oil	Plum	Papaya	Shellfish
Peas	Popcorn	Passionfruit	Soy sauce
Pomegranate	Rice milk	Peach	Sweetened fruit juice
Pumpkin	Rice/soy/hemp/protein powders	Pineapple	Synthetic sweeteners
Rhubarb	Snow peas	Raspberry	Vinegar *except apple cider vinegar*
Rutabaga	Soy beans	Rye flour	Wheat flour
Squashes *butternut, summer, onion, etc.*	Soy milk	Strawberry	Yeast
Sweet potato	Spelt	Vegan butter	
Tofu	Sunflower oil	Vegan cheese	
Watercress	Sweet cherry	Whole wheat flour *in whole wheat bread and pasta*	
Zucchini	Watermelon	Wild rice	
	White potatoes		

Alkaline update

The valuations for each category are based on the latest biochemical testing of all the foods once they are digested. As a result, some of the foods that were rated alkaline in the first book have shifted to the acidic category, but on the whole these charts tally from book to book.

BODY OUT OF BALANCE?

When was the last time you felt truly fantastic—full of energy and clear-headed, boasting skin that's plump and youthful, hair that's glossy and thick, and knowing what you want out of life and achieving just that?

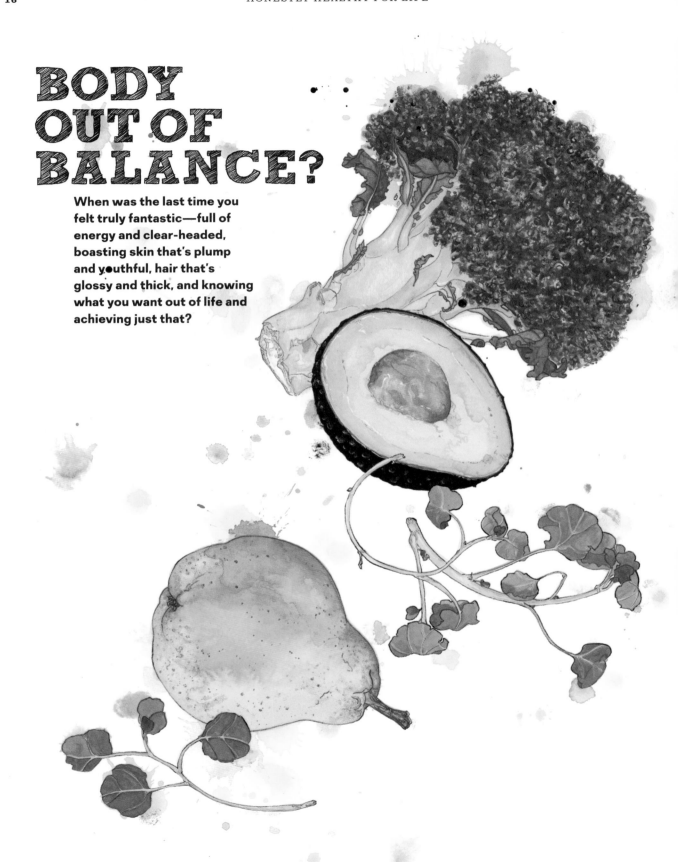

So, how are you feeling?

The optimal function of your body, and your mind for that matter, are totally dependent on getting the right balance of nutrients from your food, regular exercise, fresh air, and good-quality sleep. This should be fairly easy to achieve, and yet so many of us feel "below par" much of the time.

If you know you are not firing on all cylinders, now is the time to take stock, and look honestly at how much time you are devoting to caring for yourself. It is all too easy to run into a supermarket or café on the way to work, grabbing a quick-fix sandwich or pastry, but you already know that such a choice won't sustain you for any great length of time. Starting the day the Honestly Healthy way—with grain-based dishes, with fresh fruits and vegetables in juices and smoothies—is a whole different ball game, and one which we believe to be the first principle in alkaline eating.

Turn to page 64 to see how quick and easy it is to make your own green smoothie in the morning. This super-fast meal (they take less than five minutes to make) will provide you with a far richer source of essential nutrients, along with combating any acidity in the stomach that may have built up overnight, and supporting your body in its natural detoxification processes. A great start to any day.

Alkaline eating—whatever your age

Youth is an extraordinary gift, yet so many people take it for granted until they look back on it years later. We like to encourage everyone, at all ages, to start eating alkaline as young as possible. With the accelerating incidence of childhood obesity, it's important that parents teach their children from a young age to adopt an alkaline eating policy in the home, to ensure that at least half of what their children are consuming is predominantly healthy, fresh, and alkaline. With the lack of education for kids to learn how to cook, this is a perfect opportunity to bring good food, prepared from scratch, back into the home, and encourage your children to learn to cook. Their moods, performance at school, concentration, and ability to sleep soundly are all affected by the foods and snacks they consume. Attention deficit and hyperactive behavior have become almost pandemic, as consumption of fake foods and drinks increases, replacing fresh fruit and vegetables both at school and at home.

Make a difference in your child's life by introducing the whole household to alkaline foods—you will enhance the calm in your home, and ensure that a greater understanding of how foods affect mood and behavior is given to your children. While you can't avoid the rollercoaster of hormones that inevitably occurs during childhood and puberty, you can help to reduce the amount of acne attacks, nail-biting, and lank greasy hair that so often accompanies the teens (which are all attributable to consumption of certain foods).

Likewise, much older people need better-quality nutrition, and eating alkaline will certainly ensure that they are optimally nourished and not listless, grumpy, or forgetful. Research now shows conclusively that the incidence of age-related diseases, such as Alzheimer's, can be significantly reduced with a proper intake of antioxidants, most of which are found in the fresh, alkaline vegetables and fruit, as well as some of the vegetarian sources of protein.

What your body is trying to tell you

To ascertain just how out of balance your own body really is, we invite you to look at the following checklist that highlights the most commonly met symptoms of a body ravaged by acid-forming foods and not enough time spent giving it TLC. Even though this visual checklist isn't styled in a "from 1 to 10" format, you will quickly discover how unbalanced your body is as you work your way through the list. It's time to take stock!

 As you go through the following list, make a note of all the symptoms you identify with, as it's an ideal way of seeing just how much your health is improved when you have been following the alkaline eating program for a few weeks and then come back to check again. You will be surprised how many of the symptoms you have already forgotten you had!

Skin

- ○ Dry, flaking scalp
- ○ Irritable skin on eyelids
- ○ Subcutaneous spots on face, arms, or legs
- ○ Oily skin
- ○ Eczema
- ○ Psoriasis
- ○ Acne
- ○ Hormone-related skin changes
- ○ Flushing of skin on face and neck
- ○ Premature wrinkles
- ○ Stretch marks
- ○ Cellulite

Hair

- ○ Sudden or dramatic loss of hair (on head)
- ○ Clumps of hair falling out
- ○ Excessively greasy
- ○ Dry or brittle hair or hair that breaks easily, is lank or lack-luster

Digestive system

- ○ Burping
- ○ Coated tongue
- ○ Yellow tongue
- ○ Ulcers on tongue or gums
- ○ Acidic taste in the mouth
- ○ Bad breath
- ○ Heartburn
- ○ Indigestion
- ○ Bloating
- ○ Gas
- ○ Constipation
- ○ Diarrhea
- ○ Irritable bowel
- ○ Hemorrhoids
- ○ Itchy bottom
- ○ Frequent vomiting
- ○ Food intolerances and allergies

Nails (hands and feet)

- ○ Dry
- ○ Brittle
- ○ Splitting across the ends of the nails
- ○ Fungal infections
- ○ Raised from nail bed
- ○ Ridged, slow-growing

Energy and sleep

- ○ Lowered energy throughout the day
- ○ Fatigue
- ○ Muscle aches and pains
- ○ Broken sleep patterns; tired upon rising
- ○ Waking throughout the night
- ○ Inability to fall back to sleep
- ○ Slow to rise
- ○ Feeling unwell for no reason

Immunity
O Frequent bouts of colds and flu
O Viral infections such as shingles
O Chronic fatigue syndrome
O Slow to recover from any illness
O Frequent lung infections
O Asthma and other allergies
O Hayfever
O Frequent cystitis

Fertility
O Irregular periods
O Heavy periods
O Polycystic ovary syndrome (PCOS)
O Premenstrual syndrome
O Difficulty conceiving
O Inability to maintain a pregnancy

Mood
O "Foggy" brain
O Low mood
O Lack of motivation
O Loss of "drive"
O Frequently feeling "blue"
O Lack of self-esteem
O Irritability
O Low tolerance of others
O Feeling angry
O Crying frequently
O Inability to cope
O Anxiety
O Panic attacks

Concentration and focus
O Frequent memory loss
O Difficulty maintaining focus
O Lack of recall
O Stammering

Cardiovascular system
O Palpitations
O High blood pressure
O Shortness of breath
O Difficulty climbing stairs
O Cholesterol bags under the eyes
O Overweight
O Varicose veins
O Thread veins

Risk of diabetes?
O Addicted to sugary foods
O Frequent thirst
O Craving salt
O Frequent urination
O Suffering from PCOS
O Urinary tract infections
O Intermittent fatigue
O Tired after eating

How did your body stand up?
So, do any of these complaints sound familiar? Have you stopped even noticing certain ones? We hope that by looking through these lists you are able to identify which are the main areas of imbalance in your body. It's important to understand that these symptoms are appearing as a wake-up call from your body, and now you need to know how to address them appropriately. On the next pages, we look at each of the systems or body functions and explain why your body is behaving in this way and how alkaline eating can help to get it back on track. Bet you can't wait to turn the page!

So, what's going on on the inside?

We believe that all imbalances start with poor digestion. The digestive tract is our interface with the outside world, and how our body reacts to certain foods almost immediately is a sign of how effective our immune system is in protecting us from pathogens in the environment—and that includes our food supply. Much scientific research has shown that we have a "second brain" within the digestive system. We feel this close connection between brain and gut when we experience "butterflies in the tummy," but it has also been shown to be linked with our mood and mental state—easy to imagine when you discover that over 90% of the body's serotonin receptor sites lie in the gut. This second brain alerts us in a multitude of ways when we eat something that is either nourishing (such as fruits, vegetables, and whole grains, which elicits a sense of pleasure and well-being) or potentially damaging (foods that prompt

a reaction, from a swollen tongue to anaphylaxis).

But as we continue to consume ever more processed foods, the more our bodies attempt to adapt to the onslaught of sugars, sweeteners, additives, and preservatives, leading to lowered immunity in the gut. And with at least 70% of our immune system sitting within the digestive system, you can see the instant correlation between eating badly and feeling unwell.

While we are not suggesting that changing to an alkaline way of eating will cure any or all of the symptoms on the previous pages, you may find that many niggling problems that you have suffered from for years simply disappear as you change your eating habits from predominantly animal-based to a more vegetarian approach, eating seasonally, and in tune with nature.

So, let's take a look at the different symptoms to discover why you may be experiencing them.

Digestive system

Without a doubt, the digestive system is both complicated and miraculous in its function. It can break down everything we eat into a collection of building blocks (proteins), energy providers (carbohydrates), and other useful and vital molecules (fats). However, the present-day Western diet (which consists of an average of over 40% animal-based produce on a daily basis) creates much acidity in the body, forcing the liver, gallbladder, and intestines (and the kidneys to boot) to work far harder than is required when eating a predominantly vegetarian, alkaline diet. Countless research has now shown unequivocally that vegetarian eating helps prevent early death.

Most animal-based produce, including all meats, cow's dairy, poultry, and eggs are highly acid-forming (see page 15) and so require greater levels of digestive enzymes and hydrochloric acid in the stomach, taking far longer to be broken down as they pass along the digestive tract. Some animal foods can take several days to pass through the whole system, causing putrefaction, gas, and

bloating. That said, we include eggs in several of our recipes—while they are on the acid-forming end of the scale, they should be counted as part of the 30% of acid-forming foods in our diet as they are abundantly rich in virtually all nutrients needed for optimum nutrition.

What's more, when animal-based foods reside in the gut to this extent, the balance of "good" and "bad" bacteria—whose functions are vital in the large intestine—is disrupted, causing a wide range of symptoms including headaches and migraines, loss of concentration and focus, dry, itchy skin, eczema, and other skin irritations.

Candida microorganisms, which are found naturally in the large intestine, feed on sugars, including those found in milk-based products, such as yogurt and cheese. *Candida* can become pathogenic (harmful) if not kept in check as it can transmute into a yeast or fungal form, causing a wide range of symptoms including headaches, foggy brain or lack of concentration, bloating, gas, and feelings of general malaise.

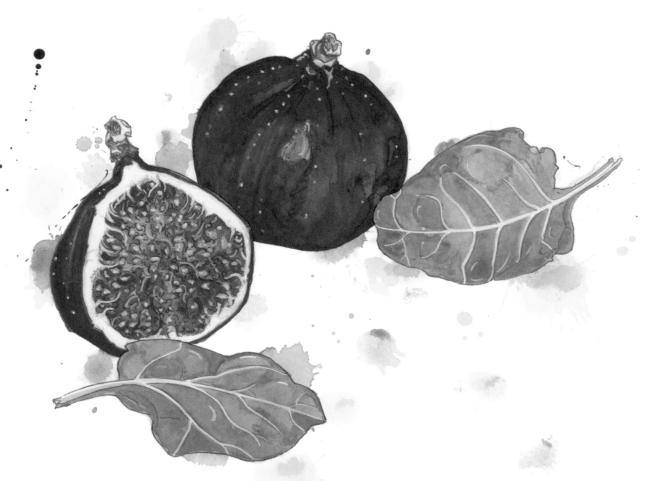

People are now finding that their sensitivities to a greater number of foods is increasing, due mainly to genetic modification of frequently consumed foods and the inclusion of pesticides and other chemicals. The digestive system cannot cope with the increased number of chemical, fake, and adulterated foods. The lining of your digestive tract allows the passage of small molecules from the gut into the bloodstream (its permeability), for transport around the body. An overgrowth of bacteria in the gut affects gut permeability and is now recognized as being a genuine cause of food intolerances and allergies, allowing particles of undigested foods to pass into the bloodstream. The fact that these particles are then carried all around the body explains why such wide-ranging symptoms can be caused by food intolerances; intolerance testing to identify the offending foods is key to getting to the bottom of the problem. Taking probiotic supplements daily can help to rebalance an upset digestive system as you identify which foods you should be omitting.

Constipation is a major cause of feeling unwell. Eating plenty of fiber from vegetables and fruit is essential to hydrate the large intestine, allowing the waste matter to travel freely through the bowel. There are two types of fiber—soluble and insoluble—and it's the soluble fiber found in fruits and vegetables, flax seeds, oats, barley, and rye that can help soften stools and make them easier to pass.

Drinking a normal amount of water for optimum hydration is essential, but drinking excessive amounts of water doesn't necessarily help the problem, as it only serves to dilute valuable digestive enzymes in the stomach and small intestine. Instead, choose to drink plenty of vegetable juices or green smoothies (see page 64) that are packed with nutrients to ensure correct hydration and mineral balance in the gut.

Skin

Your skin is the largest organ in your body, enveloping all the vital organs and structure within and providing a breathable barrier to the outside world. It is also a major organ of detoxification, allowing waste matter to be excreted through sweat glands and pores. Skin that is choked up, spotty, and congested is a strong indication that you are eating the wrong foods and your body is out of balance. The worst offenders are fried foods (including packaged snacks), red meat, processed dairy produce, and high-fat foods in the diet.

By contrast, dry skin problems are an indication of a lack of essential fats, found in nuts, seeds, and their oils. Many of our recipes include these vital foods as vegetarians can't rely on oily fish for their omega-3 essential fats, and must find them instead from nuts and seeds in particular. We love chia seeds from South America, now also grown elsewhere in the world, for their super-rich vegetarian source of anti-inflammatory omega-3 essential fats (see also the box on the right). Bulging with goodness, these hardy seeds contain up to 15 times their weight in fluids, making them a perfect hydrating food that nourishes the intestines and supplies the skin, brain, heart and, in fact, the whole body with their oils.

Eating a diet rich in highly acid-forming foods destroys some of the protective benefits provided by these essential fats, and results in inflammation, high cholesterol levels, and damaged, broken skin. But following an alkaline eating regime plumps up the skin, boosts collagen production, and protects the skin's integrity, ensuring that this miraculous barrier remains intact and healthy.

Vegetarian sources of omega-3 fats

- olives and olive oil
- chia seeds
- walnuts and walnut oil
- flax seeds and flax seed oil
- sesame seeds and sesame seed paste
- pumpkin seeds and pumpkin oil
- pecans
- pine nuts
- purslane
- wheatgerm
- green beans
- kale
- strawberries

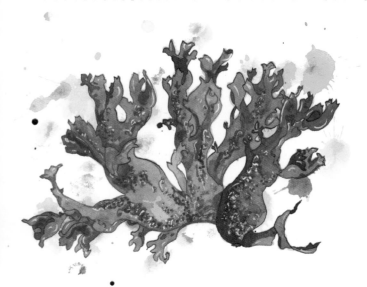

Hair

It is said that our hair is a direct indication of how healthy we are on the inside, as the shaft of the hair itself stores a record of all the toxins, heavy metals, and nutrients, and is able to be assessed by a number of tests. Even without the insult of chemical dyes and other highly toxic hair products, the hair's strength and luster is directly related to the consumption of healthy (or unhealthy) foods. Changing to an alkaline eating approach will be reflected in the hair growth within a matter of months. Silica, a mineral found in many vegetables and certain seaweeds (such as nori, wakame, and dulse), and biotin (found in whole grains, such

Nails

The strength and condition of your nails (both on the hands and on the feet) say as much about your overall health as the state of your hair, skin, or the color and texture of your tongue! The nail consists mainly of the tough protein keratin, and low-protein diets may compromise the strength and shapes of the nail. If nails are misshapen, or yellowing, this could indicate a fungal infection originating from the digestive system, such as *Candida albicans*. Lowering your intake of sugars, refined foods, and processed carbohydrates such as bread, pasta, and white rice (all of which feed any overgrowth of *Candida*), will have a beneficial effect on your nails (as well as your weight and energy levels).

Ridged nails can be a symptom of prolonged stress or a thyroid problem, particularly if they are also slow-growing, which can be a reflection of a person's slow metabolism. Since the thyroid gland regulates metabolism, supporting this hormone-producing gland can boost nail health. Eating plenty of magnesium-rich green leafy vegetables and zinc-rich foods, such as brown rice, nuts, and seeds, will help feed the thyroid's nutritional needs.

Alternatively, if your nails tend to split across the width of the nails, this could indicate poor mineral absorption and lowered stomach acid. To counter this, slow your eating; chewing your food well is a must, as well as taking a broad-spectrum digestive enzyme supplement (one that includes protease, lactase, lipase, and amylase) to improve the breakdown of your foods for better absorption of nutrients.

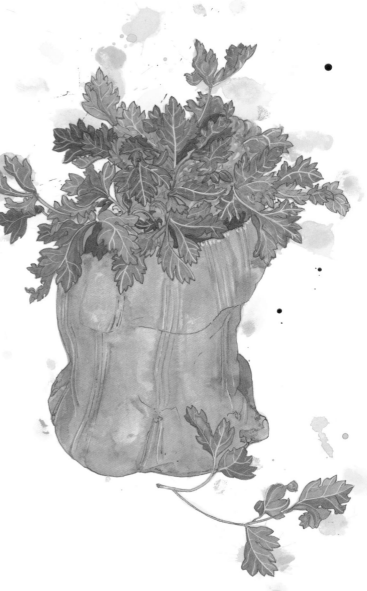

as barley, buckwheat, millet, and brown rice) are vital components of the hair shaft and hair follicle (where the hair grows from), which also requires ample essential fats to feed the developing shaft.

While other external factors, such as stress, smoking, alcohol, and environmental toxins, do affect the strength and condition of your hair, you can go a long way towards repairing damage and weakened hair and gaining your hair's natural healthy luster by adopting a more alkaline approach to nutrition.

Energy

For your body to make energy, you need all three food groups (proteins, fats, and carbohydrates), but the body favors carbohydrates as its primary source of fuel. This is the reason why so many people declare that they "can't live without pasta, potatoes (chips and fries), and cereals." Such foods are what we call "simple" carbohydrates, as they have been processed to a point where there is little nutritional value, and supply only a short burst of energy, hence the need for ever more. Our recipes, on the other hand, select the "complex" carbohydrates, derived from whole grains, since these all contain abundant nutrients (see Spinach and Carrot Muffins, page 194, and Lentil Falafel, page 219), as well as provide long-lasting energy.

It's no real surprise to discover that the top "energy drainers" are the caffeinated, processed sodas, excessive coffee and tea, and highly sweetened snacks and treats that are so abundantly available. While you know this at heart, it is sometimes difficult to pass them up, as they all have an addictive quality to them. Interestingly, they are also highly acid-forming, and challenge the liver and kidneys to dispense with them as soon as possible, thereby creating cravings for more of the same. This vicious cycle needs to be broken, and we encourage you to increase the amount of alkaline fresh foods and mineral-rich juices and smoothies in order to help you break the habits. By making this simple change, your body will feel more nourished and your energy levels will soar.

Immunity

We rely on our complex immune system to protect us from bacteria and viruses that seem to be more prevalent than ever before. Frequent travel on trains, planes, and public transportation exposes us to an ever-increasing amount of toxins, not to mention those potentially found in our processed foods and mass-produced livestock. As the majority of the immune system is actually found in the digestive tract (rather than in the bloodstream, as so many assume), what you put in your mouth has a direct effect on the support or challenge to your body's overall immunity.

Excessive amounts of alcohol, caffeinated drinks, and highly processed and fried foods are the major challenges, with sugars being the number one assault on immunity. Avoiding refined sugars and commercial sweet foods doesn't mean you can't have treats. Just a flick through the recipe section will show you that there's no shortage of healthy and naturally sweetened snacks and desserts (see Velvety Bounty Bars, page 212, and Raw Banoffee Pie, page 171). But one thing to bear in mind is that such

treats do use better-quality ingredients.

The natural forms of sweeteners you'll find within the recipe section, including date and maple syrups (preferably organic to ensure purity), cinnamon, nutmeg, and vanilla, all have beneficial properties to reduce inflammation and support immunity, rather than destroying it (see also Smarter Sweeteners, page 32).

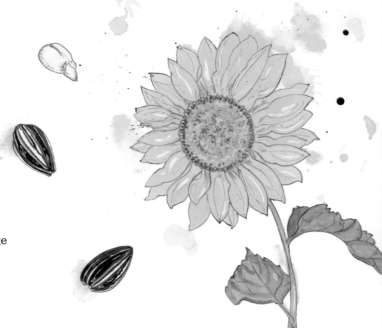

Fertility

Eating alkaline is beneficial for fertility as the body functions best when in an alkaline state. There is never a more important time for optimal nutrition than when planning a pregnancy. Fertility rates have dropped measurably in the last 15 years, as the amounts of pesticides, hormones, and antibiotics fed to livestock and the consumption of processed foods have risen exponentially with the growth of the world's population. Those antibiotics and hormones have got into the food chain and, sadly, can now be found in much of the soil on our planet.

We believe that eating organic foods as much as possible is key to your health and potential fertility. Remember that the foods you choose are the building blocks of the repair of your own body, and you need to know that you are in peak health before getting pregnant, rather than once you have discovered that you are. That said, it's never too late to start eating healthily and more mindfully.

Men's sperm count and quality (which is directly affected by food choices and stress levels) has declined in the Western world. Zinc is one of the most important minerals for the healthy production and mobility of sperm, and such micronutrients are often farmed out of the soil in commercially produced grains, such as wheat. This is why you'll notice that many breakfast cereals and breads have essential vitamins and minerals "added" to them, as those very nutrients have been processed out of such grains in the first place. Choosing organic whole grains, such as oats, rye, buckwheat, and brown rice for making breads, cakes, and cookies, is by far the healthier option (see Bircher Muesli, page 103, and Nutty Banana Muffins, page 98, as perfect examples). You'll find that not only are they easy to make, but they are also far tastier and much more satisfying.

Concentration and focus

There's nothing more frustrating than wanting to stick with a project you have started and simply not having the concentration and focus to do so. Feeding your brain requires providing it with the very matter that 60% of it is made up from—fat! But the right kind of fat is essential for providing the chemical signals, or neurotransmitters, that make those vital and myriad connections, feeding our creativity, imagination, retained knowledge, and speed of thought. In adult terms, you probably experience this toward the latter part of your day when staring at the computer but not getting anything accomplished and feeling a bit irritable. And you may well see it in your children who rush out of school having not eaten enough high-good-fat foods throughout the day and are grumpy and tetchy. We *need* good fats to function.

Essential fats (omega-3, -6 and -9) have to be derived from our diet, as we can't make them in our bodies—in alkaline eating, these are found most abundantly in nuts and seeds, with nut butters and nut and seed oils also providing excellent sources of omega nutrition. Many people mistakenly avoid these foods, believing them to be fattening, without understanding that they actually nourish the brain (and, of course, the skin).

Eating what we call the "fatty" fats—deep-fried foods, chips, pretzels, and roasted nuts—actually interferes with, or blocks, the uptake of essential fats. We challenge you to eat a small supply of nuts and seeds (or their products) on a daily basis for three weeks, and see if you don't notice your concentration and focus rise—and, of course, without having put on any weight. In fact, it is these essential fats that help you to lose stored fat! So, what are you waiting for?

Mood

It is estimated that by 2020 depression will be the second most disabling disease after heart disease in the Western world, with women being twice as likely to develop depression as men. Think back to the explanation of "the second brain" (see page 20) and you can understand why what we put into our digestive systems has such a profound effect on our moods. With most of the body's serotonin receptor sites being found in the gut, rather than in the brain itself, it becomes clear that nourishing ourselves with fresh, predominantly alkaline food has a marked effect on our mental health as well as our physical health.

While we don't suggest that good food can take the place of medication in severe cases, an alkaline diet can go a long way to maintaining good mood, balanced self-esteem, and emotional calm. You have only to stop drinking coffee for a couple of weeks to witness the loss of agitation and anxiety that may well have been an accepted part of your life for years. Many people are now choosing "detox"-style holidays or retreats, as they become increasingly aware that their daily consumption may be affecting their mood. For the same reasons that you need essential fats for concentration and focus, you also need the full range of B vitamins (see page 39) as well as a good supply of protein to balance levels of the serotonin and dopamine neurotransmitters in the brain.

All food sourced from animals, including goat's and sheep's cheese, and eggs of all types,

contains complete proteins. But for the vegan, it is necessary to find the non-vegetarian sources. Plant protein is found in anything that grows substantially larger than its original self. Think sunflower seeds into flowers, or walnuts and almonds into trees. It is the protein that allows them to grow and, once eaten, such proteins are broken down into the building blocks of amino acids, which can be easily utilized by our brains and bodies. These amino acids supply the neurotransmitters with the fuel to fire, and any deficiency will inevitably affect your mood.

Vitamin B3, or niacin as it is also known, is the predominant vitamin associated with low mood and depression. Animal produce contains the richest sources of vitamin B3, so eating eggs in a predominantly vegetarian program is a good way of ensuring your diet has enough of this vitamin; as we mentioned before, eggs are high on the acid-forming scale but are a rich source of niacin and so form part of the 30% daily allocation of acid-forming foods. But other good vegetarian sources of niacin include nutritional yeast (see Chocolate Kale Chips page 84), rice bran (which is a great alternative to wheat bran), most whole grains (such as buckwheat, quinoa, and rye) and sundried tomatoes, which can be rehydrated to bring out their full nutritional potential.

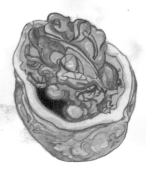

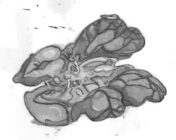

Cardiovascular health

The link between animal-based, acid-forming foods and heart disease is becoming ever more apparent: as these foods are high in saturated fat, cholesterol, and trans fats (such as those found in margarine, deep-fried foods, and baked goods cooked at high temperatures), leading to deposits in the arteries, which cause raised blood pressure and increase the risk of stroke. Healthy arteries, and indeed the heart muscle itself, is dependent on a variety of nutrients—including essential fats found in nuts and seeds and their oils, which also have an anti-inflammatory effect.

Vitamin C has a neutralizing effect on any arterial plaque (what doctors call the deposits that build up within the arteries), keeping blood flowing smoothly and the arteries clear and healthy. Vitamin C is a water-soluble vitamin, so we need to consume vitamin C-rich foods on a daily basis as we cannot store it in the body. Berries, peppers, tomatoes, sweet potatoes, squashes, and pumpkin are all excellent sources of vitamin C. Vitamin C works in conjunction with vitamin E, another powerful antioxidant vitamin, found most predominantly in avocados, pine nuts, almonds, sunflower seeds, and olives. So, to maximize

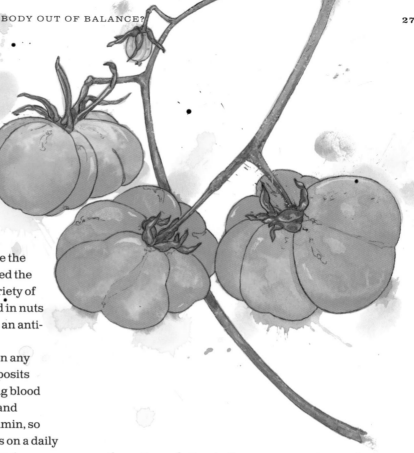

the actions of vitamin C, ensure you eat enough foods rich in vitamin E, too. The Mediterranean approach to eating has long been considered one of the most heart-healthy approaches to eating, as the use of nuts, oils, and fresh, brightly colored fruit and vegetables are at the center of its ethos, which also aligns with the alkaline approach.

Risk of diabetes?

Type 2 diabetes (what is also called late-onset diabetes and is caused by poor dietary choices and obesity) is one of the fastest-growing health issues in the Western world; it's hardly surprising, though, when you realize just how many people are consuming a highly processed, simple-carbohydrate-based diet. We believe that our alkaline way of eating, based on the combination of complex carbohydrates, vegetarian protein, and essential fats is the single most effective way of preventing the likelihood of developing this massively inhibiting condition.

Chromium-rich foods optimize insulin production (insulin is the hormone that allows glucose into all the cells of the body; see also page 29), thereby ensuring balanced blood sugar levels and regulating energy levels throughout the day. Chromium-rich foods fall in both the alkaline and the acid-forming camps, and it is wise to ensure you eat enough foods from both sources of this essential blood-sugar-regulating micronutrient. Organic eggs, broccoli, sweet potato, apple, tomato, and whole grains, such as rye, barley, brown rice, and millet, contain some of the richest sources of this essential mineral.

BALANCING TRICKS

Much is written in nutritional features and books—and even daily newspapers—about the importance of balancing your blood sugar levels, but what does this actually mean? At the end of the last section (see page 27), we addressed how to avoid type 2 diabetes through the regular consumption of foods rich in chromium, which supports insulin production. But to understand how best to balance your blood sugar levels, let's first look at the basics of how insulin works.

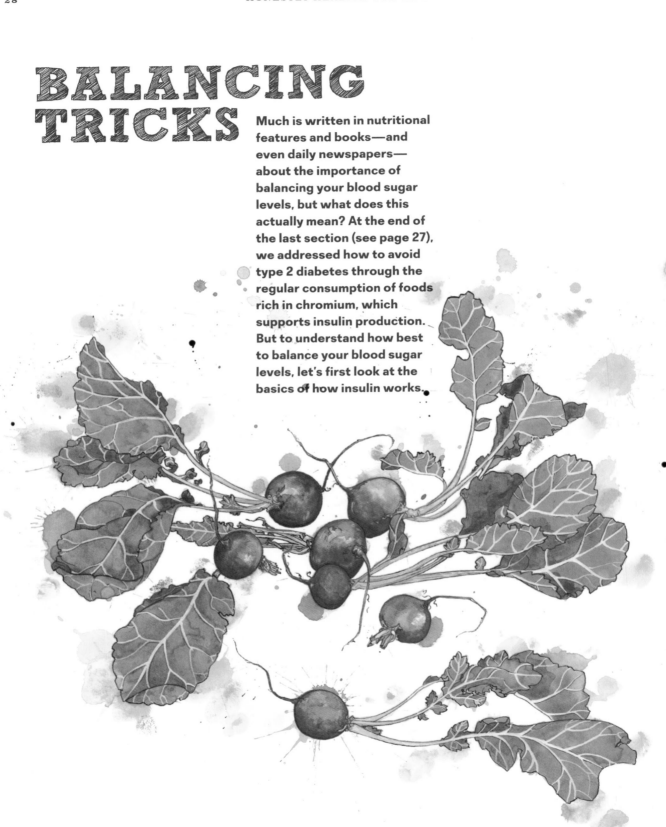

How insulin works

As we've mentioned before, your body likes to have a good supply of carbohydrates (its preferred fuel source) so that it can be broken down into a basic sugar (glucose), ready for transporting in the blood all over the body. But how does this sugar get from your bloodstream into all the cells that need energy? The answer is: with the help of a vital partner—the hormone insulin.

Insulin is produced in the pancreas, a slender, leaf-shaped organ that sits beneath the stomach and is found behind the left front ribcage. Insulin is essential for unlocking access to deliver essential nutrients into the body's cells—think of it like a key that opens a door for glucose to power all their cellular processes, thereby keeping you energized and ready for anything. If glucose remains in the bloodstream, the cells can't access this potential energy source and your body and brain will soon start to feel tired and unable to function properly.

The pancreas carefully matches the production of insulin to mirror the levels of glucose in the blood. It is essential that the level of glucose in the blood is not raised too quickly, as this would pre-empt a state of diabetes, and it is the role of insulin to regulate the levels of glucose in the bloodstream on a moment-to-moment basis. When you eat too many refined carbohydrates, sweeteners, and processed foods, this delicate balance in the bloodstream is challenged, and

the pancreas has a greater demand put upon it to regulate the blood glucose levels. When this challenge occurs on a daily basis, the pancreas cannot keep up with the demand for insulin production, resulting in what we call "insulin resistance" or Syndrome X as it is now known, in which glucose remains in the bloodstream where it's unable to be accessed by the body's cells. The pancreas's delicate balancing act can be disrupted by additional factors, such as stress, toxins in the gut or bloodstream, and the regular consumption of processed foods, as well as drinking caffeinated drinks to "keep going" when you're tired or exhausted (and that's no surprise).

The body's natural adaptive mechanisms will only shut down when the pancreas can no longer respond at the speed required by the demands on it, resulting in an inability to function—this shutdown is known as the diabetic state, and can be devastating to anyone who experiences it. It can also be life-threatening.

The blood sugar rollercoaster—don't get on

The fluctuations of blood sugar levels occur naturally throughout the day as the food you eat is broken down into glucose and transported to where it is needed (brain, muscles, heart, lungs, etc.). However, providing you eat regularly throughout the day and don't skip meals, these fluctuations are negligible. Our snack recipes are high in slow-releasing sugars that help stabilize blood sugar throughout the day, rather than sugar-rich convenience foods that push the blood sugar levels up fast but let them plummet soon afterward. Snacking is good. If you don't eat for many hours at a time, you will notice your concentration and focus diminish as well as feeling irritable and fatigued. I always use the analogy of the steam engine—if you don't keep the fire stoked, the train will slow down and ultimately stop!

The essentials of balance

Many people live on pre-packaged, processed foods that have added sugars and preservatives that directly interfere with insulin production. Think of the average daily Western diet—commercial cereals, white bread sandwiches, and pasta dishes that are both economical and quick to make at home. But you have to ask yourself—how much energy am I getting from such foods? While they may be filling or even temporarily satisfying, do they provide you with the nutrients you need to produce energy at a cellular level? The answer is inevitably "no," as you seek more of the same, in increasing doses, throughout the day. The typical diet of bagels for breakfast, sandwiches for lunch, cookies or chips for snacks, and pasta for supper does little more than increase the waistline, rather than nourishing the body and mind. This is not what we'd call eating, it is merely "stuffing" or "filling" and it is one of the fastest routes towards developing type 2 diabetes. The combination of sugars and highly processed grains (usually wheat) repeatedly raises blood sugar levels, demanding an immediate response from the pancreas to pump out yet more insulin—this is what can trigger type 2 diabetes.

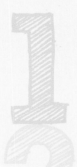

The optimal way of supporting the pancreas's balancing act is threefold:

1 to consume some protein (vegetarian or animal) with each meal

2 to eat on a regular basis

3 to avoid synthetic or processed sugars that inevitably disrupt the production of insulin.

The ideal way to nourish the body's energy-producing powerhouses, balance blood sugar levels, and appropriately place demands on insulin production is as follows:

❤ Make sure that each meal, and mini-meal, contains a source of complex carbohydrates, such as oats, rye, brown rice, or quinoa, to provide a form of slow-release energy.

❤ Add some protein, such as legumes, beans, nuts, seeds, or a choice of organic soy produce, such as tofu or tempeh.

❤ Combine a selection of fresh vegetables or fruits to provide an excellent source of fiber and antioxidants.

❤ Finish with a source of essential fats, such as olive oil or sunflower oil in a dressing (see page 82) or a sprinkling of toasted seeds to top a salad or soup.

The combination of complex carbohydrates with protein is the best coupling of foods, as protein takes longer to digest than grains, ensuring the energy derived from them is released slowly—thereby stabilizing blood sugar levels over a longer period of time. For example, in the Puy Lentil, Brown Rice, and Sweet Potato Salad (see page 70), the lentils provide protein while the rice offers the complex carbohydrate. Such a combination is both satisfying and filling.

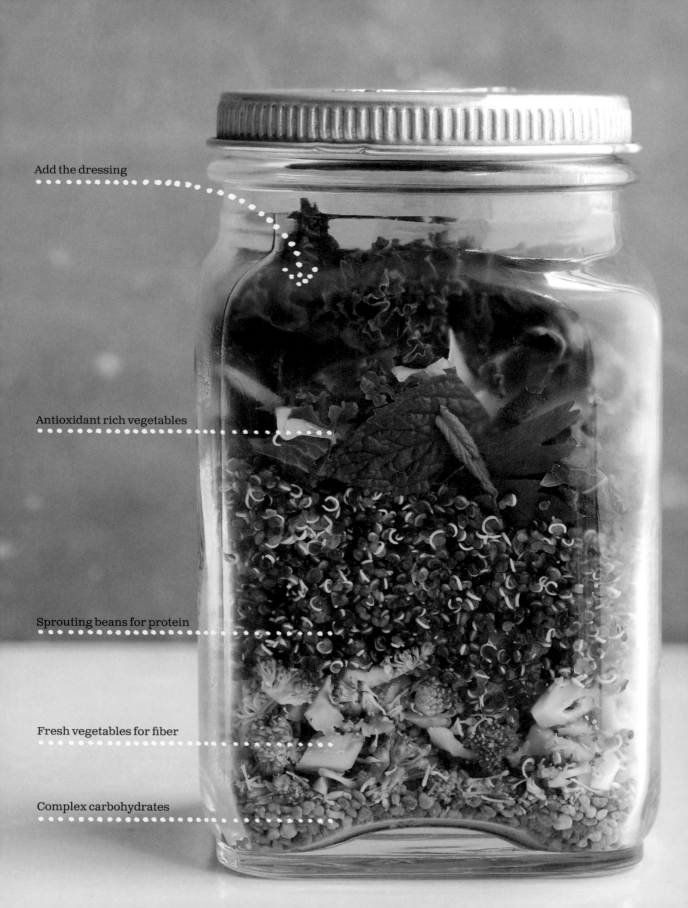

Add the dressing

Antioxidant rich vegetables

Sprouting beans for protein

Fresh vegetables for fiber

Complex carbohydrates

Eat more often

Eating on a regular basis is the second most important ideal for balancing your blood sugar levels—many people skip meals during the day, "saving" their eating for their evening meal. While you might believe this to be a smart trick to control your weight, in fact the opposite is true! When your blood sugar levels drop as a result of nothing having been eaten, and insulin production is under-challenged, the body responds by slowing down the metabolic rate, believing it to be in a state of starvation. Far better, then, to eat no less than every three hours, with three main meals and two snacks in between to ensure improved mood, energy and focus (see also pages 44–45).

The notion that eating only once or twice a day will suffice merely confuses the body as to where it should be deriving its energy, and it will look to burning up its own lean body mass as a source of fuel. This approach may work for those that are aiming to lose weight, but will wreak havoc on their concentration and mood in the process.

SMARTER SWEETENERS

You'll find a range of sugar alternatives used in the recipe section, including these below.

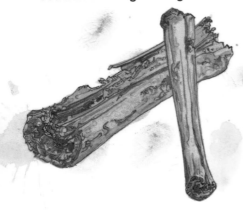

Cinnamon The bark of the cinnamon tree was once highly prized for trading in the Caribbean and rightly so. As a natural sweetener, it helps to regulate blood sugar levels, supporting the production of insulin. It also has anti-inflammatory properties, helping to calm an inflamed gut, and prevents bloating. Cinnamon is a perfect sweetener for baking and poaching, whether in its original stick form or ground into a fine powder.

Nutmeg This nut from the nutmeg tree, native to several islands in Indonesia, has a warm and spicy aroma. Again, it was a valuable commodity historically, and was traded around the world. Nutmeg is known to have anti-fungal and digestive properties, as well as being a rich source of copper, calcium, manganese, and potassium. While not as sweet as cinnamon, its spicy sweet flavor works well with brassica vegetables (such as cabbage and Chinese cabbage), as well as in homemade cakes, cookies, and breads. It's ideally stored in its whole nut form—simply grate it as you need it.

Vanilla Vanilla beans are the sun-dried seed pod of a climbing orchid. The vanilla flowers are pollinated by hand and along with its lengthy drying time, this labor-intensive process yields a highly prized and expensive ingredient. It's mainly grown in Madagascar, Mexico, and Tahiti. Whether you choose to buy vanilla beans or vanilla extract, buy the best that you can afford to impart your baking with the soft, sweet flavor of this wonderfully fragrant ingredient.

Coconut palm sugar This natural sweetener is as sweet as sugar, but more nutritious. It is made from the nectar or sap of the coconut palm tree. Although it is super-sweet, it has a low glycemic index and so works in harmony with blood sugar. To avoid getting hooked on its sweetness, we recommend only using it in small amounts. In terms of sourcing this sweetener, look for organic and unprocessed versions; check that it's pure coconut palm sugar.

Umeboshi plum purée This sweet condiment is used extensively in Japanese cuisine and has many health benefits. It is made by slowly pickling the ume fruit in salt, and then extracting the purée that results from the breakdown and fermenting of the fruit. Many cheap versions have been dyed and processed, so be selective when buying and choose a Japanese version. The taste is tart and tangy, but it is very alkalizing in the body; the Japanese frequently start their day, or a meal, by eating two umeboshi plums, or add it to soft rice, as a cure-all when treating sickness or loss of appetite.

Pomegranate molasses This thick, dark syrup is a concentrated form of pomegranate juice. It is sweet but also sharp and fruity, and so can be used instead of vinegar or lemon juice as well as a sweetener. It should be used sparingly as it contains a lot of sugars (glucose and fructose, among others).

Manuka honey This honey is traditionally produced only in New Zealand, where bees feed on the native manuka bushes. Its immunity-enhancing properties are renowned—from wound-healing to virus-preventing—but it is vital that you purchase the genuine version only. Use sparingly, as this honey, like all honeys, is very high in glucose and so can affect blood sugar levels.

For those who are aiming for improved mood, energy, and focus, eating three main meals a day, with one or two snacks in between is still the best approach to maintaining blood sugar levels.

Sugars and sweeteners

There is a plethora of information regarding sugar alternatives and, at Honestly Healthy, we want to make sure that any sweet tastes used in our recipes are derived from the purest sources possible. Let's be very clear here—refined sugar, in all forms, be it white, brown, or dark brown, is not good for you! While sugar cane (the source of all refined sugars) is a natural source, the final product you buy is highly processed, with all fiber removed, thereby wreaking havoc on your blood sugar levels, your blood cholesterol levels, and your waistline. Pure and simple—don't use sugar.

Sweetness is a taste, though, that many of us enjoy and so seek it out as one of the five tastes to create a balance. So, it's good to know that there are healthier alternatives available (see below).

Maple syrup This syrup is actually the sap from the maple tree—slashes are cut in the bark of the tree and the sap (or syrup) is collected as it oozes out. Native Americans have long used it as a medicine as well as a food. It is a fantastic source of zinc, and may help to regulate cholesterol levels, which other sugars cannot claim. Zinc is also vital for the immune system, so a good-quality maple syrup is infinitely preferable to any other sugar source. All maple syrups are graded and we recommend going for the best; it may be more expensive but it has a more subtle taste and is less processed.

Date syrup The date palm tree has been growing for millennia and dates are ancient fruits. This natural syrup is a super-concentrated form of dates; it is a mixture of glucose and fructose, but is also a good source of vitamin C and vitamin B1 and B2. Care should be taken to source organic date syrup to ensure that it has not been overprocessed.

Brown rice syrup Derived from ground brown rice, consisting of 43% maltose and 3% fructose, this natural sweetener has a low glycemic index (its GI is only 26). Be sure to choose an organic version of this syrup.

Yacon syrup This dark golden-brown syrup is derived from the tuber of the yacon plant, which is found in the Andes regions of South America; the initial liquid is evaporated to create a thick syrup. Like other natural sweeteners, yacon syrup has a low glycemic index, and so doesn't create sugar highs and lows in the bloodstream, like refined sugars do.

Xylitol Extracted from hardwood trees and the fibers of some fruits and vegetables, xylitol is a sugar alcohol. This natural sweetener contains far fewer calories than processed cane sugar and, like coconut palm sugar (opposite), has a low glycemic index, therefore it doesn't send blood sugar levels on a rollercoaster ride. It does, however, have a slight after-taste that some people find unpalatable. You can use it as a sugar substitute but it can make baked goodies a bit crumbly.

Agave syrup Also known as agave nectar, agave syrup is derived from the blue weber agave plant and is sweeter than refined sugar. We recommend you buy organic raw agave (rather than the cheaper, processed alternatives) and always use it in small quantities. Like yacon syrup and xylitol, it also has a low glycemic index; it's 39 (anything below 55 on this index is considered low), which means that it affects your blood sugar balance far less than any refined cane sugar does.

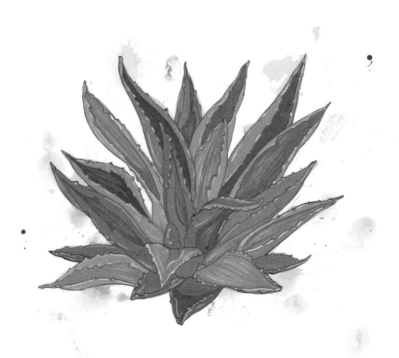

Weighing up the ingredients

Choose smart carbohydrates

Often considered the "foe" for those that are aiming to lose weight, collectively carbohydrates are the most important foods required for producing energy. Complex carbohydrates are the whole grains (such as buckwheat, oats, rye, millet, and teff) as well as all fruits and vegetables.

Simple carbohydrates, on the other hand, are those grains that have been hulled, washed, bleached, and otherwise processed to produce the fine white flour found in bagels, cookies, and buns.

THE TRUTH ABOUT GLUTEN

The majority of all commercially produced cereals, breads, cookies, and cakes are derived from processed wheat flour, as it is a strong flour due to its high gluten content. Gluten is actually Latin for "glue," so it's no surprise that this ingredient can aggravate the gut lining in some people. It behaves like a wallpaper paste when combined with the digestive juices and enzymes in the gut, preventing the absorption of essential vitamins and minerals. In severe cases, those who are allergic to gluten may develop celiac disease or inflammatory gut reactions.

Gluten is not just found in wheat, though; it's also found in rye, barley, and oats, but to a far lesser extent. What's more, these grains are rarely processed to the extent that wheat is, so they can be tolerated by most people. Fortunately, gluten-free oats are readily available for those who really can't tolerate an iota of gluten. For most, the amount of gluten found in rye and barley is rarely damaging, and these grains make excellent substitutes for wheat when making breads and cakes.

Even though these carbohydrates might taste fine, they have actually had most of their goodness and nourishment wrung out of them. So their "taste" has been artificially created through the use of a plethora of additives and sweeteners.

Our Honestly Healthy recipes use only whole grains as these are ultimately far more delicious and provide your body with the nutrients it needs. So, make the smart move now and switch to making complex carbohydrates part of every meal—your body and your mind will thank you for it.

Get to know your proteins

The word protein comes from the Greek word "protos," meaning "first things." Proteins in turn are made from the building blocks of amino acids, some of which our bodies can manufacture (the so called non-essential amino acids) and some of which they can't (essential amino acids, see right). It's interesting to note that 75% of the solid parts of your body are made up from protein, which forms the building blocks as well as repairing material. If you don't eat enough protein, the body literally breaks down faster than it is being rebuilt—a situation known as catabolism—and is found most profoundly in cases of starvation.

All animal proteins are considered "complete proteins," as they contain all eight essential amino acids the body requires for rebuilding and repair. In vegetarian eating, it is the combination of legumes, beans, and grains that achieve all eight amino acids, with the only vegetarian source of complete protein being soy produce. (However, a word of caution here, as much of the soy products available today are derived from genetically modified soy beans, we believe that consumption of soy products should be restricted to only once or twice a week. And what's more, you should make an effort to find organically produced soy derivatives, such as tofu, tempeh, and soy sauce or tamari (wheat-free soy sauce).)

Unless you are vegan, you can best derive your essential amino acids from goat's and sheep's milk and cheeses, eggs of all types (chicken, duck, and quail—the latter of which when boiled make a great

WHAT ARE THE ESSENTIAL AMINO ACIDS?

As we've mentioned already, there are eight essential amino acids that our body can't make itself so we have to source them through the foods we eat. See the chart below for how to eat to ensure you have the full complement.

AMINO ACID	ESSENTIAL FOR	FOUND IN
PHENYLALANINE	creating insulin and helping to regulate blood sugar levels; the structure of collagen and elastin in the skin	eggs, organic soy produce, and seaweed and algae products
TRYPTOPHAN	maintaining mental function and clarity through its conversion into serotonin; aiding good sleep; the production of serotonin; regulating and elevating mood	eggs, nuts, bananas, and seaweed and algae products
LYSINE	the absorption of calcium from other foods; the integrity of skin; for energy production in muscles at a cellular level (in conjunction with methionine)	eggs, mung beans, chickpeas, hazelnuts, and seaweed and algae products
METHIONINE	supporting the immune system in prevention of allergies; the production of serotonin to regulate mood and produce relaxation	sunflower seeds, avocados, and seaweed and algae products
LEUCINE, ISOLEUCINE AND VALINE	wound healing; the rebuilding and repair of muscles	all nuts and seeds and seaweed and algae products
THREONINE	supporting the immune system; reducing/controlling inflammation, such as in eczema, arthritis, and irritable bowel syndrome; the production of collagen and elastin to support the integrity of the skin	ricotta, wheatgerm, oat-germ, and seaweed and algae products

snack to carry with you when out and about). If you are vegan, then eating a good complement of nuts and seeds, beans, and legumes is essential, together with organic sources of soy-based products, such as tempeh and tofu (see Peppered Tofu BBQ Skewers, page 186, and Sienna's Spaghetti Bolognaise, page 135). In addition, seaweeds and algae products provide the broadest range of essential amino acids (see above).

A lack of protein in the diet ultimately compromises all our body's and brain's functions and is often found to be at the root of depression itself. Take note, then, how most of the recipes adhere to the combination of protein with complex carbohydrates to ensure the delivery of all essential amino acids when eating alkaline.

Opt for healthy fats

We have already mentioned the role of essential fats (see page 25), explaining that we require these fats for optimal brain function, breaking down stored fat, and ensuring that the arteries don't become clogged with deposits of saturated fat (found in cow's dairy produce, red meat, and poultry).

Lesser known is the fact that all hormones are created from the essential fats (including insulin, see page 29), and every cell in your body requires these fats for their outer layer of protection. You can observe people on a low-fat, no-fat diet, as their skin becomes crepey and fine, losing its elasticity (often prematurely), as their skin cells are starved of these essential nutrients. In nutritional practice, we always look to the skin to assess whether or not a person's essential fatty acid status is balanced.

Most importantly, the same essential fats are required for a healthy heart and circulation, as they ensure the integrity of the arterial walls and help to reduce the damage caused by ingesting saturated and trans fats.

For those who eat fish, essential omega fats are consumed in the form of oily fish. While vegetarians look to the omega-3 fats in seeds and nuts (and their oils). The supreme sources of omega-3 fats are chia seeds, quinoa, and sesame seeds—all of which can be ground, cooked at a low temperature, or made into seed butters, such as sesame seed butter (tahini). In addition, omega-3 fats are anti-inflammatory as well as being highly hydrating to the skin.

Omega-6 and -9 essential fats are also found in the same foods as omega-3 fats, contributing to hormone production and nerve transmission from brain to body. Eating such foods regularly will also contribute to a well-functioning digestive system. Soaking nuts and seeds in water for a few hours before eating or using in a recipe helps to make them more digestible to those who sometimes complain of indigestion.

Saturated fats, found in all animal produce, including cow's dairy (cream, ice cream, milk, and cheeses) block the role of the essential fats—you can see this in those who eat a lot of red meat, fried foods, and deep-fried snacks as their skin is more lined, and apparently ravaged, as they have little protection from the damage of the sun and the elements. What's more, the consumption of processed meats also severely interferes with the absorption of the essential fats, thereby having a doubly negative action on the body. What more evidence do you need to cut out (or at least cut down) on your consumption of animal produce?

The all-important micronutrients

Knowledge is power, so we feel it is important for you to know why you are eating certain foods rather than just eating what we say is healthy. Everyone knows that vegetables are good for us, but each plays a specific role in our bodies and brains, whether it's supporting immunity, repairing damage, or protecting us from external damage. So too, the grains, beans, and legumes in this book. For those of you who want to dig a little deeper, we suggest that you look at the chart on the following pages to see how foods benefit specific organs and systems in the body.

While we know that some of these foods don't appeal to everyone, it is important to recognize why "a varied diet" is so often recommended. Many people eat the same foods day in and out, resulting in obvious deficiencies. Challenge yourself to try new seasonal vegetables as they come into the market, and add one or two grains that you haven't tried before. Add also to your repertoire of beans and legumes to ensure that you are providing yourself with a wide range of amino acids for rebuilding and repair, healing, and metabolism.

Green leafy vegetables contain almost all the vitamins and minerals in the charts on pages 38–39, proving why they should form a regular part of your daily diet. This is why we include them in everything from smoothies to risottos and snacks. Don't forget that this category also includes salad leaves, such as arugula and watercress, parsley and cilantro, which are easy to add to any meal for an all-round nutrient burst.

Seeking out the new and novel

Tash and I firmly believe that a happy kitchen is one that is constantly looking for new ingredients, to keep the palate tickled and the body nourished. So, meet a couple of our new-found favorites.

Kuzu

This ancient Oriental starch is taken from the root of the kuzu plant. It is a natural thickener, which can be used in baking, custards, and desserts (see pages 107 and 136, for example). It is nutritionally rich, being harvested when the sap is fullest in the vine, is very low in calories, and doesn't upset blood sugar balance.

Chia seeds

The chia seed is grown as a grain, having originated from Mexico and Guatemala, where the Aztecs used it for its rich source of energy-producing properties. We now know that chia has the highest level of omega-3 essential fatty acids of any seed and can absorb up to 15 times its own weight in fluids, making it a marvellous source of dietary fiber. As such, it helps to lower blood cholesterol levels and balance blood sugar levels. It becomes gelatin-like in water and so is less abrasive on the digestive tract, enabling those with digestive inflammatory complaints, such as Crohn's disease, to tolerate it and even benefit from it.

Chia is also a rich source of the minerals manganese and phosphorus, essential for maintaining strong bones and teeth. It also contains tryptophan, an amino acid that is the starting block for the production of serotonin, the body's "happy hormone." Tryptophan elicits calmness and improves sleep.

What's more, chia is safe for young children to have—make into gelatin or add to smoothies—although it should be soaked for a couple of hours to allow the seed to swell first, to avoid any swelling taking place in their guts. The seeds can also be ground into a fine flour, which becomes quite gelatinous when soaked, making it an excellent vegetarian alternative to gelatin for mousses and puddings.

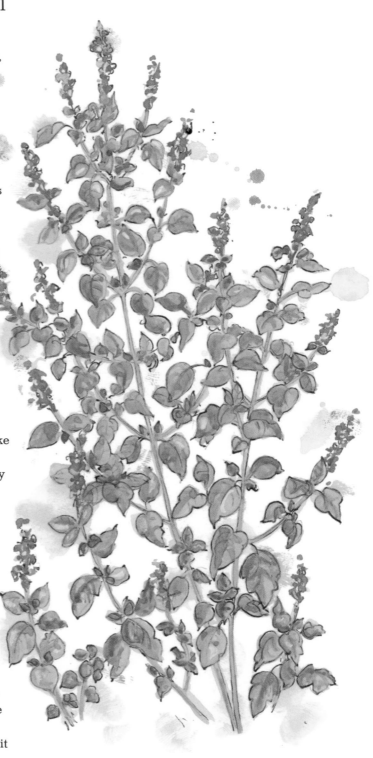

Which foods supply me with...?

MINERAL	REQUIRED FOR	FOUND IN	SIGNS OF DEFICIENCY
Calcium	building strong bones and teeth, hair and nails (in conjunction with vitamins D, C, and iron); supporting cardiovascular health; muscular contraction; a strong nervous system	almonds, and other nuts, organic soy produce (including tofu), kale, chard, Savoy cabbage, Chinese cabbage, broccoli, asparagus, globe artichokes, dairy produce, bony fish (sardines, herring, etc.), sesame seeds, and figs	muscle cramps; aching bones and muscles; teeth problems and alignment
Magnesium	relaxing muscles; cardiovascular and nervous systems; managing stress (adrenal glands); supporting metabolism (thyroid); carrying calcium into bones; relaxation and supporting sleep; aids mental clarity	citrus fruits, all green leafy vegetables (such as kale, chard, spinach, parsley, cabbage, Chinese cabbage, and watercress), carrots, tomatoes, onions, garlic, sweetcorn, almonds, hazelnuts, pecans, walnuts, and cashew nuts	muscle cramps and twitches; restless legs; fidgeting; insomnia; poor concentration; irritability; palpitations
Potassium	balancing sodium for the hydration of all the fluid content in the body; regulating metabolism at a cellular level to create energy	hazelnuts, almonds, lentils, sesame seeds, watercress, spring greens, spinach, asparagus, kiwi fruit, figs, and bananas	pins and needles in hands and feet; frequent thirst; cellulite; constipation; palpitations; low or high blood pressure
Sodium	all nerve transmissions; muscle contraction; carrying nutrients into every cell in the body, balanced by potassium	virtually all foods—naturally in all fruits and vegetables, low in nuts and seeds, high in cheeses	rarely occurs, but muscle cramps (particularly after exercise); fatigue; confusion and headache; nausea; dehydration in hot climates
Iodine	thyroid gland to produce thyroxine hormone to stimulate and regulate metabolism	all seaweed (nori, wakame, kelp), blue–green algae, seafood, and garlic	unexplained weight gain; inability to lose weight; fatigue; constipation; cold hands and feet; crying easily; lowered immunity; frequent colds and infections
Selenium	supporting the immune system and the production of natural killer cells to ward off cancers; protecting the heart and cardiovascular system; supporting liver detoxification	Brazil nuts, sunflower seeds, sesame seeds, pumpkin seeds, onions, lentils, chickpeas, black-eyed peas, and lima beans	frequent infections; slow wound healing; chronic fatigue; signs of premature aging (graying hair, wrinkled skin)
Chromium	the production of insulin; regulating blood sugar, as well as cholesterol in the liver; helping to protect the cardiovascular system	egg yolks, all nuts and seeds, barley, buckwheat, teff, millet, rye, lentils, and broccoli	irritability; sugar cravings; mood swings; premenstrual syndrome; dizziness; low energy; frequent thirst
Iron	formation of red blood cells, especially the oxygen-carrying pigment hemoglobin; carrying oxygen to the brain and muscles; immunity; growth and development throughout the body	all dark green leafy vegetables (especially watercress, parsley, kale, broccoli, and spinach), raisins, prunes, figs, dates, brown rice, and egg yolks	fatigue; anemia; muscle weakness; diarrhea; dizziness; depression; increased infections
Manganese	control of blood sugar levels and metabolism; bone health and rebuilding skin and internal tissues; hormone production; antioxidant protection against free radical damage	pumpkin seeds, sesame seeds, flax seeds, sunflower seeds, brown rice, lentils, rye, oats, buckwheat, quinoa, pecans, walnuts, hazelnuts, and macadamia nuts	irritability; dizziness; joint pains; fatigue; lowered fertility in women
Copper	the formation of red blood cells and white blood cells; the metabolism of glucose into energy (thyroid); brain function and collagen formation	sesame and sunflower seeds, cashew nuts, coconut milk, avocados, asparagus, garlic, chestnuts, mushrooms, beans, and oat bran	anemia; raised cholesterol; hair loss; poor immunity; depression
Zinc	strong immunity; efficient protein digestion; production of insulin; regulating metabolism; skin tone; wound healing; making new cells and enzymes; sperm formation	cashew nuts, pumpkin seeds, lentils, brown rice, chickpeas, buckwheat, quinoa, and tofu	stretch marks; poor wound healing; frequent viral and bacterial infections; lowered fertility; white specks on fingernails
Sulfur	the body's detoxification processes; protecting cardiovascular system; lowering cholesterol; anti-parasitic activities; production of energy at a cellular level; production of cartilage	onions, garlic, cabbage, Brussels sprouts, beans, and peas	dry skin; eczema; loss of skin elasticity; thinning hair; brittle nails; back pain, arthritis; raised cholesterol

VITAMIN	REQUIRED FOR	FOUND IN	SIGNS OF DEFICIENCY
Vitamin A (and beta-carotene found in fruits and vegetables)	strong immune system; growth and repair of bones; skin, teeth, and eye health	egg yolks, dairy produce, pumpkins and squashes, yellow and red peppers, tomatoes, apricots, peaches, mango, and papaya	dry skin and flaking nails; poor sense of smell; loss of appetite; acne; mouth ulcers; sinus problems; poor night vision; poor wound healing
Vitamin D	calcium absorption into bones and phosphate regulation; strong bones; healthy teeth; regulates body temperature; supports immunity	dairy produce and egg yolks, plus it's synthesized in the body in the presence of sunlight	misaligned teeth; aching bones and muscles; muscle weakness
Vitamin E	healthy and supple skin; immune system; cardiovascular health; reducing scarring; wrinkles	all nuts and seeds, vegetable oils, eggs, avocados, oats, rye, brown rice, and millet	dry and flaking skin; poor wound healing; eczema; shortness of breath and palpitations; anemia; fatigue
Vitamin K	vitamin D to work properly in bone building and repair; blood-clotting factors; preventing heavy menstrual bleeding	live yogurt and other dairy produce, egg yolks, all dark green leafy vegetables (such as kale, chard, spinach, and cabbage), pumpkin seed oil, and sunflower seed oil	easy bruising; heavy periods; osteoporosis
Thiamin— vitamin B1	digestion of carbohydrates; production of energy; cardiovascular health; supporting nervous system; mental clarity; memory	eggs, whole grains including rye, millet, buckwheat, oats and quinoa, beans, peas, and legumes	depression; poor memory and concentration; lethargy and fatigue; headaches; pain and noise sensitivity; indigestion
Riboflavin— vitamin B2	digestion and metabolism of all proteins, fats, and carbohydrates; healthy skin, hair, and nails; managing stress	dairy produce, yogurt, brown rice, kale, cabbage, watercress, and spinach	digestive problems; diarrhea; constipation; dizziness; insomnia; poor concentration; chapped lips; watery eyes; scaly skin around nose, ears, and mouth
Niacin— vitamin B3	production of sex hormones; thyroxine to regulate metabolism; insulin for regulation of blood sugar levels and energy; keeping digestive system healthy; regulating mood; healthy nervous system	brown rice, millet, oats, buckwheat, quinoa, egg yolks, dairy produce, and dark green leafy vegetables	lowered sexual drive, performance and fertility; irritability and fatigue; lack of motivation and concentration; insomnia; dizziness and blood sugar problems; sugar cravings
Pantothenic acid— vitamin B5	supporting adrenal glands in management of stress; metabolism of fats and carbohydrates; healthy nervous and immune system; protecting all ear, nose, and throat areas	egg yolks, wheat, rye, barley, millet, all green leafy vegetables, broccoli, and potatoes	low blood pressure; insomnia; depression; adrenal fatigue; teeth grinding; chest infections; constipation
Pyridoxine— vitamin B6	mood regulation; concentration; growth, healing, and repair; digestion and metabolism of protein into energy; formation of hemoglobin	whole grains, dairy produce, eggs, and all green leafy vegetables, such as chard, kale, cabbage, bok choi, watercress, and parsley	anemia; itchy rashes; scaly skin on the lips; cracks at the corners of the mouth; a swollen tongue; depression; confusion; a weak immune system
Cobalamin— vitamin B12	production of red blood cells; cardiovascular health; growth, repair and healing; healthy nervous system; concentration; energy release	eggs, dairy produce, and micro-algae, such as spirulina and chlorella	anemia; fatigue; restlessness; mood swings; poor concentration; confusion; depression; heart problems
Folic acid	building of antibodies for immunity; protein and carbohydrate digestion and metabolism; preventing anemia; promoting cardiovascular health; (alongside vitamin B12) production of hemoglobin	carrots, apricots, avocados, pumpkin and squashes, egg yolks, rye, millet and buckwheat, all green leafy vegetables (such as kale and spinach), Brussels sprouts, cabbage, broccoli, peas, beans, brown rice, and chilis	anemia; shortness of breath; fatigue; feeling faint
Biotin	healthy skin, hair, and nails; digestion of proteins and fats for metabolism into energy	brown rice, nuts, egg yolks, chard, carrots, almonds, walnuts, strawberries, raspberries, cucumber, and cauliflower	excessive hair loss; eczema; psoriasis; scaly skin; muscle cramps; fatigue
Vitamin C	all immunity; cardiovascular health; development of sex hormones; managing stress (adrenals); effective wound healing; maintenance of connective tissues; protection against viral and bacterial infections	all citrus fruits, kiwis, watermelon, red berries, blackcurrants, Brussels sprouts, squashes and pumpkin, sweet peppers, cabbage, broccoli, cauliflower, potatoes, and spinach	frequent infections; poor wound healing; skin problems; fatigue; depression; easy bruising; bleeding gums; varicose veins

FROM UPGRADING TO FIRST CLASS

In our first book (*Eating the Alkaline Way*), we introduced the concept of "upgrading," that is, making small changes to your eating habits to create a significant change to your energy levels, mood, and general health. For example, upgrading from white rice to brown rice, or from high-sugar breakfast cereal to muesli or porridge, which provides you with far more nutrients and far fewer additives.

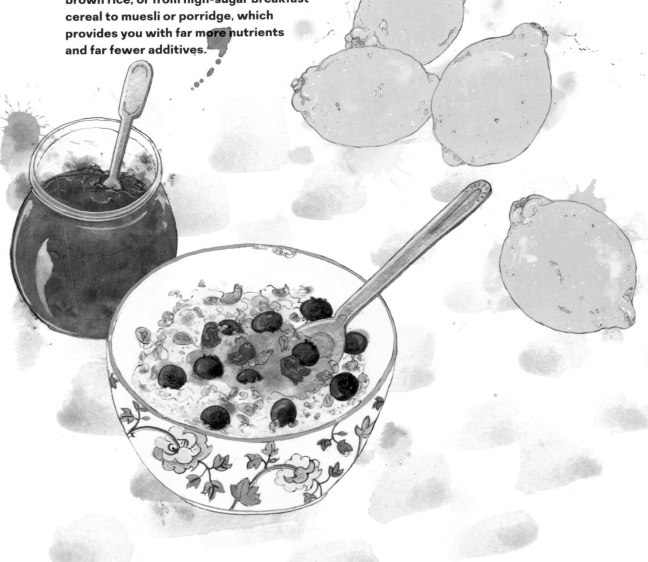

Such upgrading is a step-by-step process and needn't all be done at once. It's inevitable that, as you improve your choices, you will search for ever-increasing nutrient-rich foods and start experimenting with those. As you will see from the recipes section, Tash has used her creativity in the kitchen to make delicious dishes out of lesser-known ingredients for both their alkalinity and their nourishing properties (for example, Chestnut Tart, page 201, Easy Edamame Dip, page 211, and Chia Seed Porridge, page 63). This is what we call "first class" eating. Not to suggest that it is more expensive, but rather that it provides you with a far greater range of nutrients, from foods not stripped of their natural goodness.

If this is the first Honestly Healthy book you have bought, you may want to get the original book to go through the five-day Cleanse and then the Lifestyle plan, which invites you to follow the 70:30 alkaline:acid ratio of foods for everyday eating.

Onwards and upwards

For those readers coming here after following the Cleanse in our first book and who are now following the Lifestyle plan, you will probably have already completely changed what you stock in your pantry, where you buy your food from, and what you cook and eat (and what you simply never eat any more).

For all readers—new and devoted—what you'll discover within the pages of this book are myriad recipes to help you continue to live the Honestly Healthy lifestyle while still fitting in all the usual life events, celebrations ,and entertaining possibilities. Whether you're putting on a kid's birthday party, want to make on-the-go lunches, or just want ideas for a lazy Sunday breakfast, the recipe section has something to fit every bill.

What do you want to achieve?

Many people have goals and targets—be that alleviating physical symptoms, a special event in your life for which you want to look and feel your best or, more generally, a whole new chapter in your life for which you have chosen to look after yourself in a completely different way. We always recommend that everyone sets goals and timelines.

For those of you who have come to this second Honestly Healthy book without having read the first one, know that you will be challenged to give up certain foods that you may have eaten all your life—wheat-based commercial cereals, breads, and cookies (see page 34) and cow's dairy produce including milk, cream, ice cream, and cheese). You may well have never considered how these—what we call acid-forming foods—may have been the very cause of some of your symptoms or feeling generally under-par.

Keeping track

We recommend that you give up one food group before another (for instance, wheat-based foods or cow's dairy produce) rather than both at the same time, as this way you can ease yourself into alkaline eating, without worrying about what you can replace these foods with. Most importantly, keeping a note of which foods you're not eating helps you to determine any specific sensitivities that you may have; you will know all too quickly which foods cause which symptoms by omitting one group for three weeks and then reintroducing that acid-forming food group (be it wheat, cow's dairy produce, or red meat, for example) for one day—sometimes the effects can be that profound!

Keeping a food diary lets you see how certain foods affect you adversely almost immediately— stomach pains and cramps, brain fog, irritability, constipation, or diarrhea. As we outlined earlier (see pages 20–26), such symptoms are all ways your body is trying to tell you that what you're eating doesn't work for you. If you have omitted the foods for three weeks or more, the immune reaction to those foods will be quite pronounced.

The ideal situation—70:30

Some readers may have previously followed a high-protein diet, which is aimed at providing you with more energy and helps with losing weight. The major problem with this approach is that it is very acid-forming in the body, placing a heavy burden on the liver and kidneys, which have to use valuable nutrients, such as magnesium, to buffer the effects of breaking down and eliminating the acidic residues. Such an example is a high meat/chicken/fish diet with few or no fruits and vegetables, and virtually no grains at all. In Honestly Healthy terms this style of diet would put you in the bracket of 10%:90% alkaline forming foods:acid-forming foods. Not a healthy way, we feel, to feed your body or your mind.

When we recommend having a ratio of 70% alkaline to 30% acid-forming foods, we directly illustrate that it's kinder on your digestion and balances your body's functions better if you always eat a higher ratio of alkaline foods. If we look at one of the recipes, for example, The Perfect Omelet (see page 61), the simple and humble egg, which is acid-forming, is rendered far more alkaline by the inclusion of the tomato, portobello mushroom, and spinach. And you'll see plenty of green leafy vegetables and many other vegetables and salad leaves are included in almost every main meal, to ensure that you get the balance right. Check out, too, the Spirulina Protein Balls (see page 87), where the oranges and dry unsweetened coconut create a balance even in a sweet treat.

Just because a recipe or a meal on a menu has an acid-forming ingredient doesn't mean that it is to be avoided. On the contrary, it encourages you to look for the balance of vegetables and whole grains and some fruits, such as dates and apricots, to help boost a dish's alkaline status. You'll know you're on track and when you have reached your optimal target of our recommended 70%:30% alkaline foods to acid-forming foods—it'll be when your energy has returned, you can think clearly and stay focused for hours, your skin and hair look fabulous, and your friends comment that you haven't "looked this good in years."

More important than physical appearance is the list of symptoms that you complained of a few months ago. All those niggling digestive problems, skin disruption, painful or irregular periods, headaches, and migraines are long forgotten. It may be useful for you to return to the symptom checklist (see pages 18–19) to remind yourself of what improvements you may already have noticed since changing your eating habits.

In our experience, some of the first improvements in following an alkaline way of eating always seem to be in change of mood, an improved ability to cope with daily challenges, and a better quality of sleep. As your body adjusts to greatly increased absorption of vital nutrients, your hormones will rebalance themselves (including those involved in metabolism) and you will be able to lose any extra pounds that you simply couldn't shift before. With your new-found increased energy, you can exercise more efficiently, allowing your body to become more flexible as your muscles become stronger and have more stamina—whatever your form of exercise.

You may find that everything has started to grow faster—you need to visit the hairdresser more frequently, your nails need constant trimming, and the turnover of skin is greatly improved, giving you a healthy glow. Such noticeable indicators are a great reflection that your internal organs are now working optimally and your overall digestion is vastly improved, which is at the very core of well-being.

One of the most important areas of your well-being and health is your mental attitude—feeling well increases your self-esteem, as you realize you can take on anything that is thrown at you. Your new-found passion for the foods you put in your mouth has doubtless made you realize how out of control your eating habits were before or how little time you spent on nourishing yourself.

Falling off the wagon

Both Tash and I feel that you should be able to
have a little of what you love, without feeling that
this will "tip the balance" or make you feel that
you have undone all the good work to date! I was
a passionate chocoholic in my earlier life, until I
realized that it was one of the main triggers for my
migraines. I still love chocolate, but now eat only
good-quality dark chocolate, with no milk solids
or added sugars. Tash has a weakness for
cakes, and so she has found clever ways
to make healthier, yet nonetheless
delicious versions of all those she
couldn't resist! You will see how many
"treats" we have managed to include in
this book, but, as the name suggests, we
aren't suggesting that you eat these every
day—they are "treats," remember.

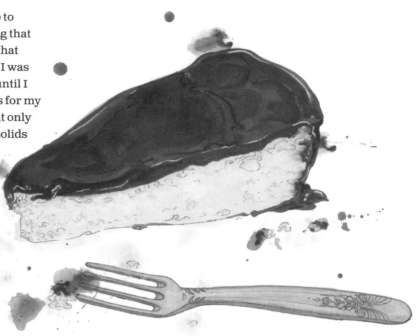

If passion becomes obsession

As with anything in life, there is a risk that some
people become slightly obsessive about how much
alkaline foods they're eating—perhaps this is the
most recent of many attempts to "go on a diet," and
they have taken it to the extreme, telling family
and friends that they "can't eat" various foods for
health reasons. While 70:30 is the ideal ratio for
alkaline:acid-forming foods, it doesn't mean that
80:20 is better, or even 90:10. Nothing done to
extremes is healthy and we feel very strongly that
life is all about balance.

    While alkaline eating does exclude certain
foods, it doesn't mean you should ever find
yourself in the position where you turn away well-
intentioned dishes that others have cooked for you.
Give yourself permission to have something that is
"off radar;" it's a great experiment to observe how

that food affects you. While such eating isn't going
to kill you or your new-found healthy eating, it does
reinforce what you have already come to know.
Simply take note of which foods your body really
no longer digests. In reality, it never could, but that
will be much clearer to you now.

    In my experience in nutritional practice
over the last 20 years with many people who have
become obsessed about their food habits, I suggest
that if you are finding that you have become too
fastidious about what is on your plate, to the point
where it is more painful than pleasurable to eat out
at restaurants or have dinner at friends' houses,
that you consider seeing a nutritionist to help you
move forward with this attitude. Eating alkaline is
not a diet, it is a way of life and as such should be—
and is—able to be adaptable.

A FIVE-DAY MENU PLANNER

To help you get an idea of what the right ratio of alkaline foods to acid-forming foods looks like, take a look at our menu planner that covers any five days of the week (see right). As you'll know by now, we recommend the optimum ratio of alkaline eating in any one day be 70:30 (alkaline:acid-forming). Almost all of the recipes fit this 70:30 rule so you can simply open the book, pick a recipe, and feel safe in the knowledge that you'll be along the right lines that day. But it's a good idea to plan a week's worth of eating so that you can get a good variety of vegetables and fruits, different grains and legumes as well as a variety of cuisines so that your palate is always tickled and you're excited about what you're eating.

Some people may prefer to follow this menu for a few weeks to get the idea of the balance of alkaline to acid-forming foods and how it makes them feel (in their body and in their mind), whereas others might like to do it just once and then dip in and out of the recipe section based on what's in their shopping basket that day or what their favorite recipes are. Others may prefer to get an idea of how it works from this chart and then pick and choose similar recipes at will.

This menu planner presents a great alkaline menu for five days and includes snacks and one weekly treat. You can obviously chop and change the menus to suit your work and play lifestyle that week. But do remember, a treat is a treat; you don't have to have one every day, or even every week—the whole point of a treat is that it is exactly that, a treat! If you go with the idea of a Sunday prep night, you'll find that making soups and tarts ahead and freezing them is massively time saving and they make great impromptu lunches and dinners—that way, you always have something to take with you or to come home to!

DAY 1

Morning
My Favorite Granola (see page 96), with sliced apple and almond milk and a good handful of fresh berries
Green Tea

Lunch
Celeriac and Orange Soup (see page 260) and a slice of Roasted Tomato and Spinach Tart (see page 240)

Evening
Raw Green Curry with Zucchini "Noodles" (see page 74) and a green salad, plus a dressing of your choice (see page 82)

Snack
Almond Berry Cake (see page 233)

DAY 4

Morning
Poached Egg and Spinach on Quinoa Toast (see page 95)
White Tea

Lunch
Salad Wraps (see page 69)

Evening
Sienna's Spaghetti Bolognaise (see page 135)

Snack
Easy Edamame Dip (see page 211) with raw crudités

DAY 2

Morning
The Perfect Omelet (see page 61) with a slice of pumpernickel toast
Fennel Tea

Lunch
Thai Mango and Corn Salad with Pomegranate Relish (see page 230)
Juice (see pages 266–267) or Green Smoothie (see page 64)

Evening
Spinach Pearl Barley "Risotto" (see page 246)

Snack
Sunflower Seed Paste (see page 88) with raw carrots and celery dippers

DAY 3

Morning
Bircher Muesli (see page 103) with sliced apricots
Green Smoothie (see page 64)

Lunch
Quinoa, Lemon Kale, and Sesame Beet Salad (see page 76)
Juice (see pages 266–267) or Green Smoothie (see page 64)

Evening
Roasted Eggplant and Mango Salsa with Black Rice Noodles (see page 242) with Tahini Dressing (see page 82)

Snack
Spirulina Protein Balls (see page 87)

DAY 5

Morning
Chia Seed Porridge (see page 63) with slivered almonds and sliced peaches
Mint Tea

Lunch
Wild Mushroom Quinoa "Risotto" (see page 132) with a beet salad, plus a dressing of your choice (see page 82)

Evening
Citrus Seaweed Salad (see page 73)

Snack
Raw Hemp Granola Bars (see page 87)

TREATS FOR THE WEEK

Choose ONE of the following:
Crunchy Toffee Popcorn
(see page 118)
Melt-in-the-Mouth Donuts
(see page 124)
Raisin Oat Cookies
(see page 148)
Sticky Toffee Pudding and Custard
(see page 136)
Gluten-free Bread and Butter Pudding
(see page 182)
Moses's "Nutella"
(see page 100)
Nutty Banana Muffins
(see page 98)

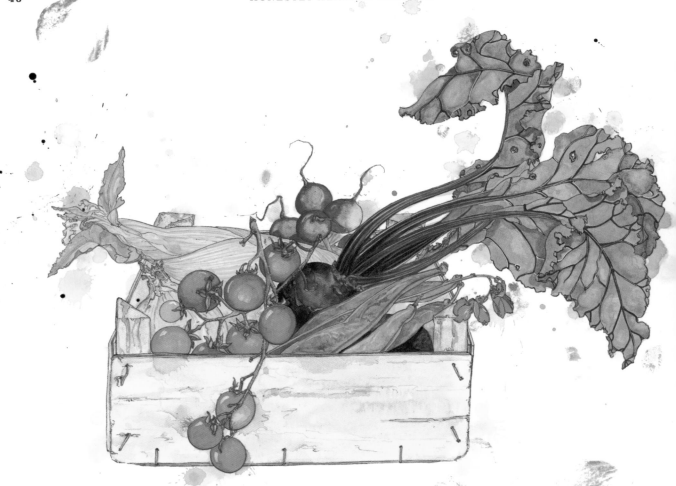

THE NEW WAY OF EATING AND COOKING

Eating the alkaline way doesn't mean simply cooking the recipes and eating the food, it's much more than that. At Honestly Healthy, we embrace alkaline eating in its entirety and that means the way you plan your menu, the ingredients you choose to buy, the way you cook, and the way you eat. As you'll discover below, becoming more aware of what you're eating and where it has come from is a worthwhile goal, and your body will thank you for it.

Eating consciously

How often do you actually sit down to your meals and think consciously about what you are eating, particularly when you are on your own? Like many people, perhaps you eat your lunch at your desk, while multi-tasking on the phone and staring at a computer screen? Or are you running around all day, grabbing a bite only when you realize how famished you are and are on your last legs? Any of these examples sound familiar?

The process of digestion starts from the moment you think about food—the thought process stimulates the production of saliva and digestive enzymes in the mouth, and the stomach is alerted to prepare for food shortly arriving. Allowing time to contemplate what you are eating and chewing your food deliberately and consciously is precisely what creates the conditions for optimal digestive function. But many people eat on the run, while they are driving or sitting on the sofa, and simply shovel the food into their mouths to satisfy a hunger in the shortest possible time—no wonder they suffer from indigestion, burping, and bloating!

Enzymes in your saliva help to start the chemical breakdown of the food as well as chewing it (which breaks it down physically), so it is important to take time to chew food until it resembles a thick liquid in the mouth. What's more, such deliberate chewing not only reduces the risk of choking, but also allows the stomach's several sets of muscles to effectively churn the food, which takes anywhere from 15 minutes to several hours, depending on the density of the food (for instance, fruit breaks down quickly, while meat takes a long time). As we age, the acidic environment of the stomach is compromised by a lowered production of hydrochloric acid, commonly resulting in indigestion. Ironically, affected people are often given antacids to reduce the discomfort.

The truth is that the symptoms for under-production and over-production of stomach acid are the same, so the medication is simply a band-aid for the problem. For everyone, we recommend taking a broad-spectrum digestive enzyme with each main meal of the day to help the stomach do its work—it's a far better and more gentle solution to a very common problem. Interestingly, too, certain medications can actually cause indigestion, so it is worth trying the digestive enzyme route, rather than taking yet more medication to rule out the causative problem of others.

We firmly believe that eating alkaline is a sure-fire way of optimizing digestive function and significantly reducing digestive complaints by ensuring that the food you eat is more easily digested and offering a nutrient-rich solution. If you have digestive problems, you will find that they inevitably improve as you increase the amount of alkaline foods in your daily diet. Try it and see for yourself. Acid-forming foods, such as cow's dairy produce, meat, and poultry, are often the direct cause of stomach and upper intestinal discomfort, and it is worth setting yourself a timeline goal to see what improves when such foods are replaced with an increased amount of vegetables and some of the more alkaline grains.

Taking time to prepare your own juices, snacks, and meals, and selecting those that you know sit well in your system, is worth its weight in gold. What you have on your plate should look appealing and have a wide range of color to create an attractive display. When eating in a restaurant, you know only too well how the presentation of the dish will delight you—it is not only for your eyes—but also to stimulate the digestive juices!

Tantalizing your tongue

The tongue is covered in thousands of papillae—think of its texture under a microscope being like a hairy bathmat—with minute projections (or taste buds) that detect both a food's taste and its texture, acting as a guide and a guard to everything you put in your mouth. There are specific areas for the five different taste categories—sweet, salty, savory (or spicy), sour, and bitter. Asian cuisines place a lot of importance on preparing dishes that provide all five tastes to ensure a harmonious balance.

Are you a sweet or savory person? Do you reach for a sugary treat or some salty nuts? The numbers of taste buds and their sensitivity have a part to play here. Some people have areas of the tongue more sensitive to sweet tastes or savory or spicy notes, which helps to shape the differences between those that have a sweet tooth and those that prefer spicy or salty foods. On average, there are between 2,000 and 8,000 papillae on an adult's tongue. As you age, these numbers decline, but they can also become damaged or desensitized through how you live your life. For instance, smoking, drinking alcohol, and chewing gum can desensitize the taste bud, and certain medications (especially those found in cancer treatments) can also impact on your ability to taste. Eating your food in its natural state, as close to nature as nature intended, will help you to develop a more taste-sensitive tongue, in turn allowing you to derive far more pleasure from the nuances of a dish with complex flavors, fresh herbs, and spices.

Tash takes great pride in developing recipes that are "layered"—that is, you can discover several different tastes as you chew the food, which reveals the different textures and flavors of a dish. Many of the recipes contain unexpected combinations of sweet and sour, where you would not usually find them together, or salty and dense, rather than salty and spicy. This element of surprise sets so many of her recipes apart—you don't get what you expect.

From the first click to the last bite

Getting organized about how you select and buy your foods is key to making sure that you have what you need in your pantry and your refrigerator. We recommend choosing a few hours during the weekend, or whenever you have time off, to prepare for the week ahead.

Farmers' markets

Both of us use the mid-week and weekend markets to select all those delicious locally grown products that often come from the smaller farms. These farmers take great care to bring their produce to market, as their livelihood depends on it. Some of these producers will have selected specialist greens and salad vegetables, or grown tree-bearing and vine-grown fruits that are derived from olden times. There's nothing like the complex tastes of older-style fruits, such as apricots, peaches, or greengages, grown in small orchards, to add to wonderful cakes and tarts (see Chestnut and Apricot Soup, page 260, and Peach and Butternut Salad, page 202).

We find this kind of food shopping far more exciting than running up and down the typical supermarket aisle, as the variety is greater and, sometimes, rather more challenging! We set ourselves targets to find the most seasonal produce and then work out different ways to play with it—it is definitely my favorite way to spend time with Tash!

Supermarket shopping

Supermarkets have their place, though, and we tend to use them for canned staples, such as ready-cooked lima beans and Puy lentils, canned tomatoes with basil, and jars of artichoke hearts and olives for emergencies. Buying such items is not a sin if it means you have a greater range of produce at your disposal. I always make sure I have a good range of different flours in stock, too. Many supermarkets now offer a good gluten-free flour range, such as gram or chickpea flour and buckwheat flour (or use an online supplier, see page 271)—with such flours to hand, you can whip up pancakes or blinis at a moment's notice.

Specialist online shopping

Order online those products that you want to store in bulk—nut milks, beans, legumes, and olive oil. Oils are always best bought in 5-quart tins where the air, light, and heat cannot get to them. Decant into beautiful dark bottles and add rosemary, sage, basil, garlic, or chili peppers to create your own selection of flavored oils. Do keep your oils away from the heat of the stove or oven—while they may be filled to the brim with antioxidants, you don't want to start a dish with a rancid oil that will make even the freshest vegetables taste foul.

We like to shop online for dried herbs and spices, but be sure to find a range that is well stored and that you don't have to buy in bulk, unless, that is, you are cooking for a massive family. Unless you are cooking in significant quantities, spices in particular lose their potency over time, even if they're stored in airtight containers, so it's better to buy a little and use that up before replenishing your supplies. Have a good clear-out of your cupboards every six months to ensure that you don't end up with dried herbs or spices that are years past their best-by date. Remember, fresh is always best, but star anise, cinnamon, allspice, and nutmeg can all be stored as these are not necessarily everyday condiments.

For the more specific ingredients, such as tamarind, mirin, and spirulina powder, simply search online. Make sure they are a reputable company for supplying such goods and will ship the products to you with appropriate packaging. Don't be seduced by cheap or cut-price products— they may be long past their best-by date. Always choose reputable brand names.

Venture into new shops

In total contrast to online shopping, Tash and I love nothing more than to find extraordinary products in Asian supermarkets and other local independent shops—some of her best dishes have been as the result of trying an ingredient that she had never encountered let alone cooked with before. So, be bold and don't be afraid to ask what something is used for traditionally— understanding how it's usually cooked or used in cooking allows you to think "outside the box" for new recipe ideas. Inspiration can be found almost every day if you embrace the possibilities.

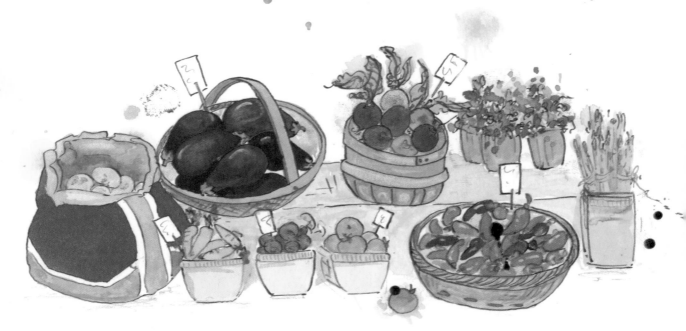

Eating raw and cooking methods

At Honestly Healthy, we love raw foods and like to cook to keep ingredients as close to their natural state as possible. But we also like the myriad possibilities cooking offers in terms of adding texture and taste. There are many ways of cooking—from roasting and baking to poaching and steaming. All have their benefits and some their drawbacks. Each of the methods below is best suited to certain ingredients to bring out the best in their taste or the texture they impart to a dish.

Eating raw—not cooking

The benefits of eating raw vegetables and fruits, or adding raw sprouted beans and seeds to salads cannot be underestimated. In this book, we have included Four Green Smoothies (see page 64) for their nutrient density, Raw Green Curry with Zucchini "Noodles" (see page 74), which uses a spiralizer to make spaghetti from fresh vegetables, and Sunflower Seed Paste or Sundried Tomato Pesto (see page 88), to name just a few. Eating raw produce delivers the highest amount of nutrients in a meal—try to include at least one juice or salad per day (even in winter) for optimal nutrition.

Dehydrating

This brilliant method of literally "drawing out the water" or fluid content of a vegetable or fruit yields a nutrient-dense, crispy version of whatever has been put into the dehydrator the night before. Dehydration isn't a quick process, which is its only downside, and dehydrated foods are a far healthier version than their commercial counterparts; this method of "cooking" is increasingly popular with the raw foodists and healthy food eaters. Some dehydrators can be reasonably priced (though some are expensive), and are a wonderful addition to any kitchen. You'll never buy chips ever again! For recipe ideas, see Fruity Roll-ups (see page 147) and Chocolate Kale Chips (see page 84).

Roasting

Roasting—using a combination of heat and oil— works amazingly well for vegetables, particularly root vegetables, as their sweetness comes through. The secret is to roast at low to medium temperatures, to ensure that there is no damage to a vegetable's nutrient values. You'll find vegetables such as butternut squash, sweet potato, beet, parsnips, and kohlrabi all roast wonderfully. For recipe ideas, see Roasted Eggplant and Mango Salsa with Black Rice Noodles (see page 242), Bejeweled Brussels Sprouts (see page 174), and Masala Roasted Root Vegetables (see page 131).

Baking

The beauty of baking is that it allows you time in the kitchen to be cooking other things while the cookies, cakes, breads, or muffins are "doing their own thing." If you think about it, baking was one of the earliest forms of cooking, when fires were constructed in pits, and foods were wrapped in dampened leaves to "bake" in the embers of the fire to allow tastes and flavors to develop, without the ingredients being overcooked.

While some may think of baking as a difficult aspect of cooking, and one that has to be incredibly precise, Tash makes it easier than you can imagine. Since she's already worked out exactly what works together, Tash combines ingredients to provide a complexity of flavors to tickle the palate. The trick with baking is to use a timer— too many cakes, cookies, and muffins are ruined because they get "forgotten" in the oven.

Blending and juicing

The ultimate tool in the Honestly Healthy kitchen is a high-speed blender (we use a Vitamix blender); we recommend that you purchase the best your money can buy. All sorts of dishes—sauces, soups, dips, dressings, and drizzles—are all pummeled together in the blender. We use ours many times a day, so the investment is actually worth it. A juicer is not the same as a blender, and all you need to look for in a juicer is one that works on a centrifugal basis, since that ensures the maximum volume of juice from your ingredients.

The benefit of being able to consume muffins, for instance, that are "good for you" is immeasurable, delivering goodness from vegetables or fruits that some family members might ordinarily shy away from. For recipe ideas, see Nutty Banana Muffins (see page 98), Raisin Oat Cookies (see page 148), Orange and Almond Cake with Orange Syrup and Chocolate Frosting (see page 161), and Gingerbread Men (see page 179).

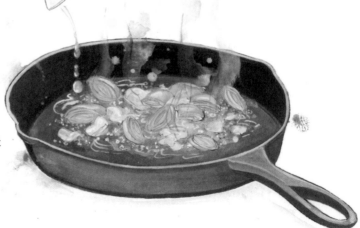

Toasting

Using the heat of an oven but without any oil, toasting is a great way of bringing out the nuttiness in granola mixes, grains, and seeds. Toasting uses low temperatures, which allows the flavors to develop without damaging the delicate essential fats found in them. Toasting barley and quinoa, in particular, if turning into risottos, can be done ahead of the actual preparation of the meal itself, and adds a wonderful depth to such dishes. For recipe ideas, see My Favorite Granola (see page 96), Orange and Aniseed Teacakes (see page 208), and Moses's "Nutella" (see page 100). All nuts and seeds can be toasted in the oven at low temperatures to prevent rancidity, and then allowed to cool completely before storing in airtight containers.

Poaching

Traditionally a cooking method used for fish, seafood, and chicken, poaching works wonderfully for soy products and vegetables to create meals-in-a-bowl, with added noodles. Ideally, the herbs, spices, and other flavors need to be poached in a water-based broth first to allow the aromas to develop before any foods are added. Ginger, lemongrass, lime leaves, chilis, and tamarind, for instance, can all meld together; the same goes for star anise, cinnamon, and nutmeg, if poaching fruits for breakfasts or puddings.

This supremely gentle way of cooking on the stove is an excellent way of preserving the shape and texture of the foods, and adding a lid keeps the aromas and nutrients contained within. For recipe ideas, see Kuzu and Berry Compôte (see page 63) and Lemongrass and Rose water Pannacotta (see page 250).

Sautéing

Cooking food in a hot pan with a little fat (butter or oil) is often used in Mediterranean cooking. We use sautéing but opt for the healthier oils, such as olive and coconut, to infuse the foods with flavor, without browning or blackening them. Sautéing allows you to "layer" flavors and cook vegetables alongside beans and legumes. Constant tossing or jiggling of the food is vital when sautéing, so do watch the pan—a minute with your back turned can result in a burned or ruined dish. The secret? It's low-temperature slow cooking. Use the juices from the pan with water and stock, reducing to intensify the flavor even more! To keep the temperature low, add splashes of water. For recipe ideas, see Lentil Falafel with Buckwheat Flatbreads (see page 219), Carrot and Zucchini Patties (see page 192), and Fennel and Leek Soup (see page 262).

Reducing

Often used in the kitchens of Michelin-starred chefs, reducing allows a combination of flavors to be simmered down to less than a third of their original volume, thereby providing a stickier consistency and a far more intense flavor. Tash tends to reduce fruits for all the delicious treats, cooking them at low temperatures to reduce them to a sticky, binding consistency. Whether savory or sweet, this is a wonderful way of producing sauces and drizzles.

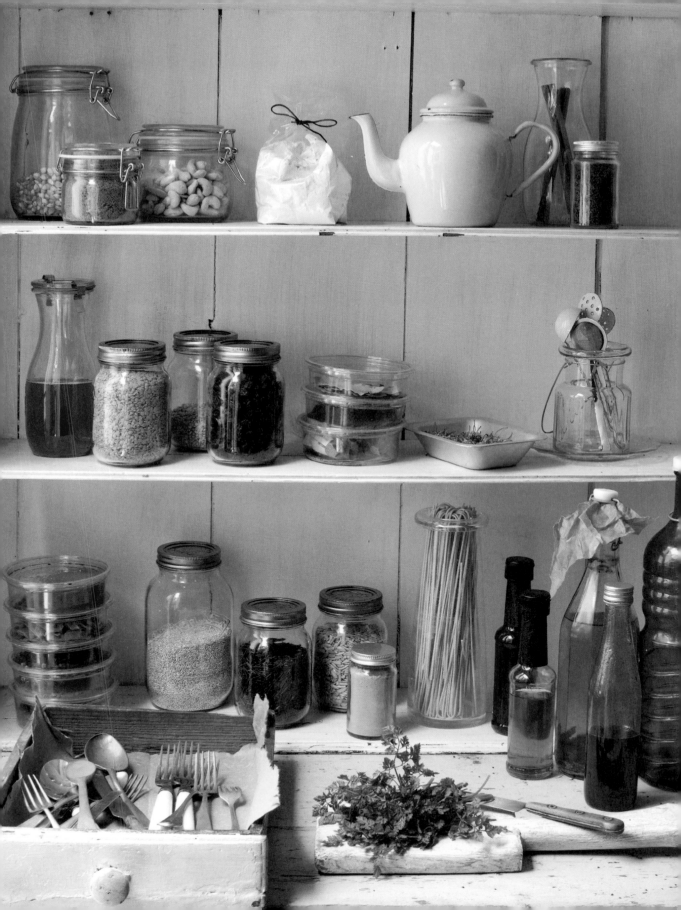

THE ULTIMATE HH PANTRY LIST

LEGUMES
Beluga lentils
Chickpeas
Lima beans
Puy lentils
Split red lentils

FLOURS
Almond
Buckwheat
Chickpea (gram)
Coconut
Cornstarch
Millet
Oat
Potato
Quinoa
Rice
Rye
Tapioca
Teff

GRAINS
Barley flakes
Brown rice (brown sushi rice, brown short-grain rice, brown basmati rice, and brown risotto rice)
Gluten-free oats
Jumbo rolled oats
Millet flakes
Pearl barley
Popcorn kernels
Red rice
Sprouted wheat
Unsweetened puffed rice
Wild rice

NUTS AND SEEDS
Almonds, whole and slivered
Aniseeds
Brazil nuts
Caraway seeds
Cashews
Chestnuts
Chia seeds
Coconuts
Fenugreek

Flax seeds
Hazelnuts
Hemp seeds
Pecans
Pine nuts
Pistachios
Poppy seeds
Pumpkin seeds
Quinoa
Sesame seeds
Sunflower seeds
Walnuts

NUT AND SEED BUTTERS
Almond
Cashew
Hazelnut
Pumpkin
Sesame seed
Sunflower

OILS
Coconut
Hemp
Olive
Pumpkin
Sunflower
Toasted sesame
Walnut

VARIOUS CONDIMENTS
Agar agar
Apple cider vinegar
Balsamic vinegar
Bouillon powder
Brown rice vinegar
Celtic sea salt
Dijon mustard
Himalayan pink salt
Mirin
Miso paste
Nutritional yeast
Orange-blossom water
Rose water
Tamari
Tamarind paste

HERBS AND SPICES
Allspice, ground
Aniseed, ground
Black onion seeds
Cayenne pepper
Celery seeds
Coriander seeds and ground
Cumin, ground
Curry powder
Dried rosemary
Fennel seeds
Fenugreek, ground
Fresh basil
Fresh bay leaf
Fresh chervil
Fresh cilantro
Fresh curry leaves (or dried)
Fresh dill
Fresh flat-leaf parsley
Fresh mint
Fresh rosemary
Fresh tarragon
Fresh thyme
Garam masala, ground
Ginger, ground
Ginger root
Horseradish, ground
Lemongrass
Mixed spice, ground
Mustard seeds
Smoked paprika
Turmeric, ground
Za'atar

NATURAL SWEETENERS
Agave powder
Agave syrup
Brown rice syrup
Cardamom
Cinnamon, ground
Coconut palm sugar
Date syrup
Dry unsweetened coconut
Manuka honey
Nutmeg
Pomegranate molasses
Raw cacao butter
Raw cacao nibs

Raw cacao powder
Star anise
Umeboshi plum purée
Vanilla extract
Vanilla bean
Xylitol

HERBAL TEAS AND COFFEE ALTERNATIVES
Barley cup
Chamomile
Dandelion coffee
Fennel
Ginger
Green tea
Jasmine
Mint
Nettle
Pu'er
Rooibos
Thyme
White tea
Yerba mate

DRIED FRUITS AND VEGETABLES
Apricots
Goji berries
Golden raisins
Kombu seaweed
Nori seaweed
Raisins
Shiitake mushrooms
Unsweetened blueberries
Unsweetened cranberries
Wakame seaweed

OTHER DRIED GOODS
Baking powder
Baking soda
Black rice noodles
Dairy-free milk powder
Gluten-free pasta
Kuzu
Xanthan gum

FRESH BUYS FROM WEEK TO WEEK

In your refrigerator

Almond milk
Coconut milk
Coconut water
Eggs
Feta
Goat's cheese
Goat's yogurt
Halloumi
Hazelnut milk
Hemp milk
Maca powder
Oat milk
Probiotic powder
Quinoa milk
Rice milk
Sheep's cheese
Smoked tofu
Soy yogurt
Spirulina
Tofu
Tofu cream cheese
Vegan butter
Wheatgrass or barley group powder

Farmers' market buys

Apples
Artichoke hearts
Arugula
Asparagus
Avocado
Bananas
Basil
Bean sprouts
Beet
Blackberries
Blueberries
Broccoli
Brussels sprouts
Cabbage
Cantaloupe
Carrots
Celeriac
Celery
Chard
Chilis
Chinese cabbage
Chives
Cilantro
Corn
Cucumber
Dates
Eggplant
Endive
Fava beans
Fennel
Figs
Flat-leaf parsley
Garlic
Ginger
Grapefruit
Grapes
Green beans
Greengages
Iceberg lettuce

Jerusalem artichokes
Kale
Kiwi
Leeks
Lemons
Limes
Mango
Mizuna
Mustard greens
Nectarine
Okra
Onions (red and white)
Oranges
Papaya
Passionfruit
Peach
Pears
Peas
Peppers (all colors)
Pineapple
Plums
Pomegranate
Porcino
Portobello mushroom
Pumpkin
Radish
Raspberries
Snow peas
Soy beans (edamame)
Spinach
Spring greens
Scallions
Squash
Strawberries
Sweet potatoes
Tomatoes
Watercress
Watermelon
Zucchini

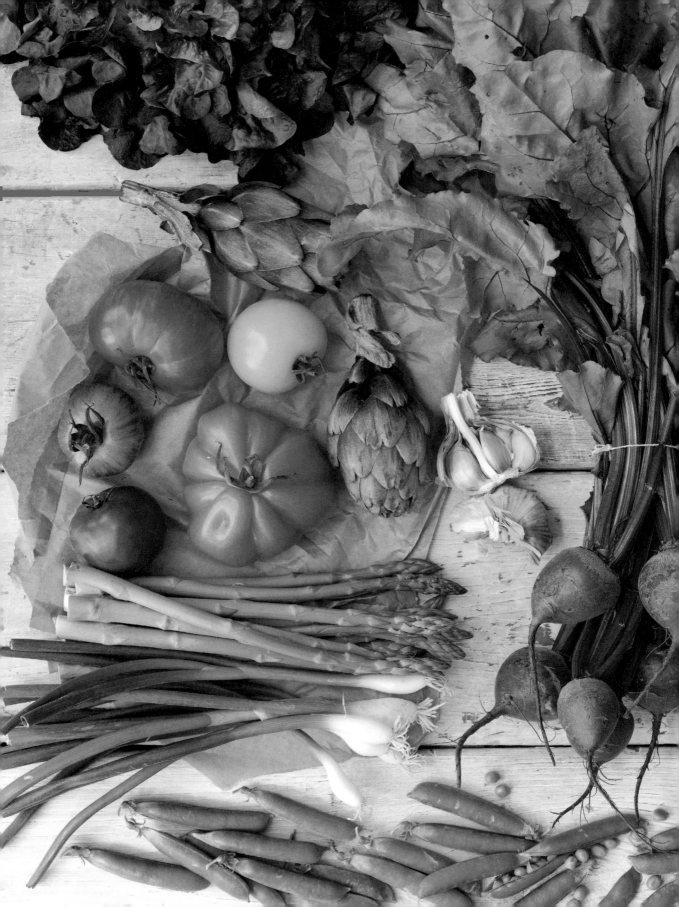

RECIPES AT A GLANCE

If you're looking for inspiration fast, then find what you want with our at-a-glance index of recipes.

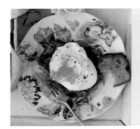

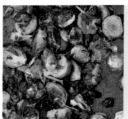

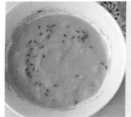

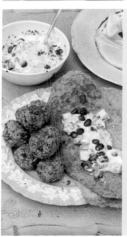

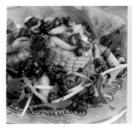

Sweet treats

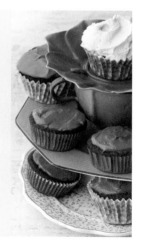

Snacks and bites

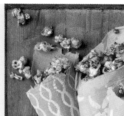

Breads and bakes

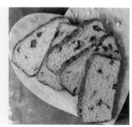

Dips, sauces, dressings, and marinades

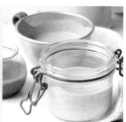

Juices

Drinks

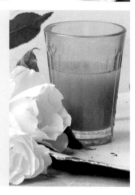

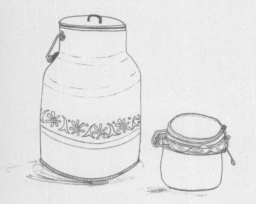

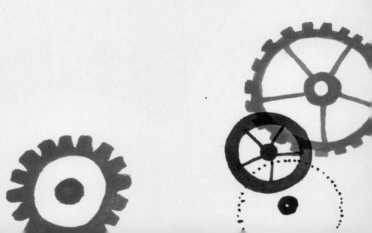

ON THE GO

This "on the go" section is to help you pre-prepare delicious and nutritious food to fit in with your busy times, so you can eat healthily and feel satisfied all of the time.

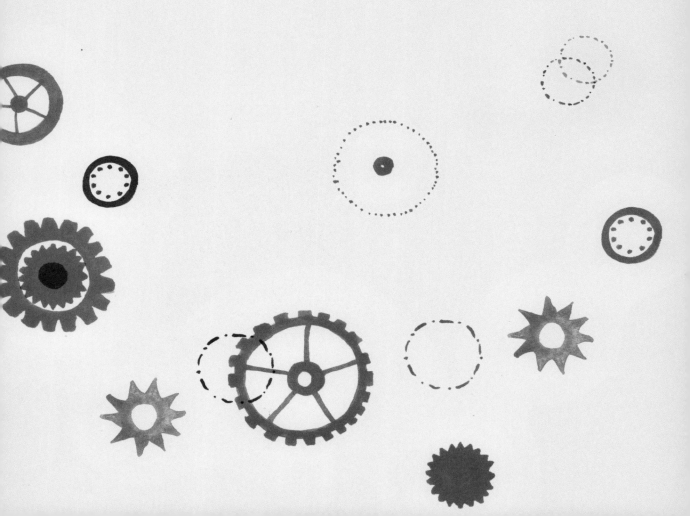

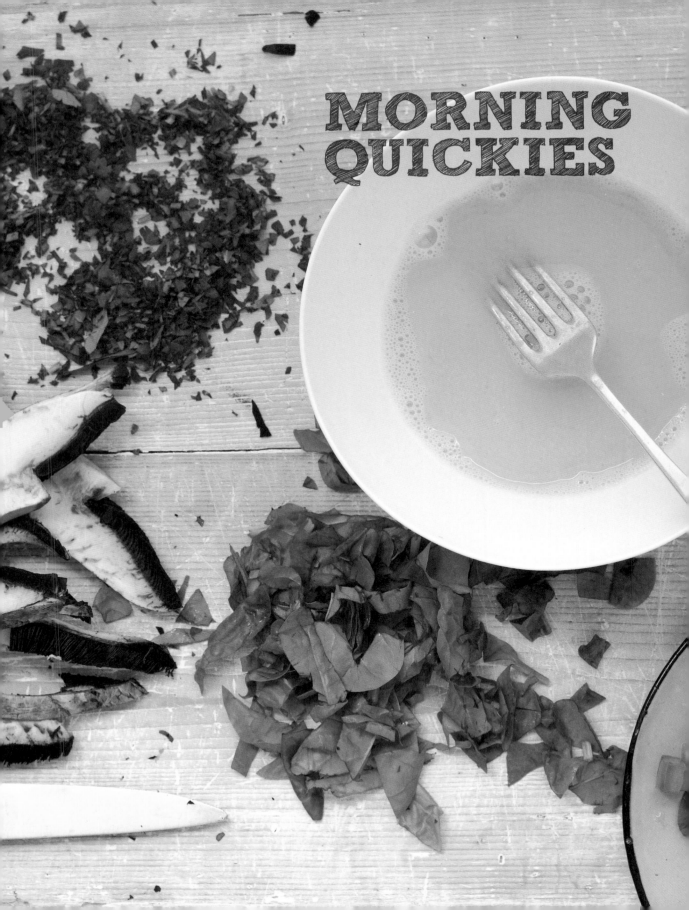

MORNING QUICKIES

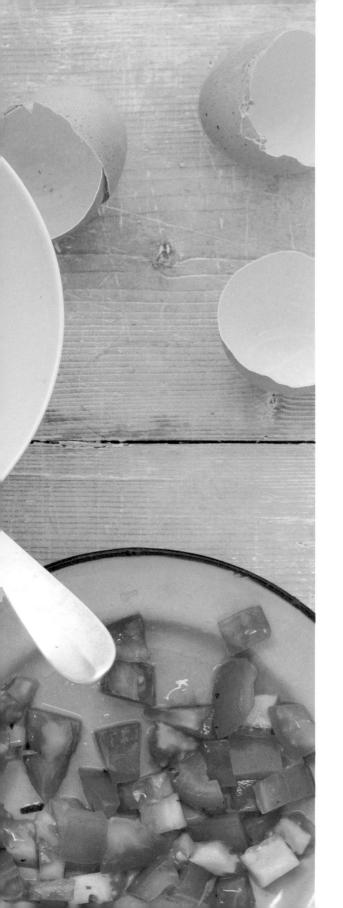

THE PERFECT OMELET

You may think making an omelet is too messy and takes too long in the mornings before work, but the more practice you have the better you'll become—especially at flipping—and the quicker you'll get.

serves 1

2 eggs

2 tbsp sunflower oil

1 large tomato, chopped

1 portobello mushroom, sliced or chopped

1¼-in chili, chopped (optional)

3 tbsp flat-leaf parsley, chopped

¼ cup baby spinach, chopped

Crack the eggs and whisk in a bowl, then set aside.

Heat 1 tablespoon of the sunflower oil in a skillet over medium heat and sauté the chopped tomato and mushroom for 2–3 minutes, until soft. Place into a separate bowl and set aside.

Wipe the skillet clean with paper towels, return to the heat, and add 1 tablespoon of sunflower oil.

Add the chili (if using) and the parsley to the egg mixture and then pour into the skillet and leave to cook for 30 seconds. Then pour the tomato and mushroom mixture onto one half of the omelet, like a half moon, and then put the chopped spinach on top of that.

If the egg will not move by gently tipping the skillet, then get a spatula and slide it under the half of the omelet without any vegetables on it. Gently and carefully flip that side over the other. Don't worry if it gets a bit messy, the look doesn't affect the taste at all—and it's going to taste delicious.

Now, for another tricky bit, flip the entire omelet over and leave to brown for another minute; you might want to use two spatulas here to help, but with practice you won't need anything but a flick of the wrist. Serve immediately and enjoy.

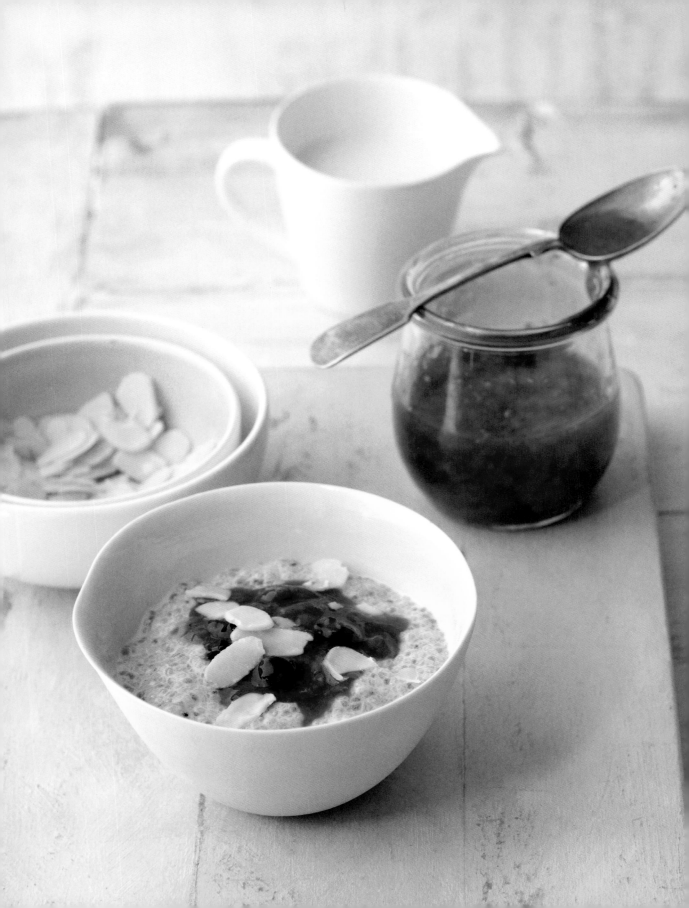

CHIA SEED PORRIDGE

With a different texture than oatmeal, this super-quick breakfast is grain-free—perfect if you are trying to steer clear of gluten or if you want to slim down. Chia seed porridge is delicious hot or cold and gives you a great start to the day; mix the flavors up by using different milk substitutes.

serves 1

3 tbsp chia seeds
1 cup almond milk
½ tsp ground cinnamon
slivered almonds, to sprinkle

Put all the ingredients except the almonds into a bowl. Stir continuously for 1 minute so that the seeds don't clump together. You can either refrigerate overnight and add a little more almond milk in the morning to loosen it up, or leave to soak for 15 minutes, sprinkle over the almonds, and then enjoy for breakfast.

Alternatively, you can move the bowl's contents into a pan and heat up gently for 3 to 5 minutes and eat warm (no need to chill overnight).

Adjust the sweetness with a little agave syrup, if needed, or garnish with fresh fruit, nuts, seeds, or even a little Kuzu and Berry Compôte (see right).

KUZU AND BERRY COMPÔTE

When you're after a sweet hit, then reach for this glorious ruby-colored compôte. It is perfect for breakfast (add to yogurt and granola, see page 96) or serve as a coulis with a cake (see page 233) for a healthy and guilt-free dessert.

makes about 2½ cups

1½ cups raspberries
1⅓ cups blackberries
2 cups water, plus 1 tbsp cold water
1 tbsp agave syrup
¼ cup kuzu
1 tsp vanilla extract

Put the berries, water, and agave syrup in a pan and bring to a simmer—this should take around 3 to 4 minutes.

Put the dried kuzu granules in a cup with 1 tablespoon of cold water, then stir until dissolved and it's become a smooth liquid.

Pour the kuzu out of the cup into the pan of hot fruit, stir well, and then take the pan off the heat. Add the vanilla extract.

Let cool (in the pan or transfer to a bowl) and then chill for an hour.

TASH'S TIPS

If you are soaking seeds overnight, you could split the quantity of chia seeds in half and replace with gluten-free oats for a more hearty option in the morning—a great alternative if you're exercising a lot.

NUTRITIONAL NUGGET

Kuzu is a natural gluten-free starch made from the Japanese kuzu root (*Pueraria lobata*). It's a thickening agent, like cornstarch or arrowroot, and is excellent at thickening all sorts of dishes, from gravy to custard. It is both easy to digest and has a soothing quality to it.

FOUR GREEN SMOOTHIES

There is no better way to start the day than with an alkalizing green smoothie. They are really filling and only take two minutes to make. So, no excuses any more not to blend one up first thing and put in a container to take to work with you. What's more, they help to keep your blood sugar levels balanced all the way to lunchtime.

Put all the ingredients into a high-speed blender and pulse. If the smoothie seems a bit too thick for your taste, simply add a little more filtered alkaline water or coconut water.

serves 1

Green Machine
1 handful spinach leaves
5-in cucumber
1 banana, peeled
2 celery stalks
½ tsp spirulina
1 cup filtered alkaline water or coconut water

Green Glorious Greens
1 handful watercress
1 pear, cored
1 head broccoli
¼ avocado
1 plum, pitted
scant ¼ cup unsweetened apple juice
1 cup filtered alkaline water or coconut water

Green Love
1 medium mango (about 6 oz), cut into cubes
⅓ cup flat-leaf parsley
1 handful kale or spinach leaves
1 tbsp flax seeds or chia seeds
1 cup filtered alkaline water or coconut water
½ apple, cored

Green Glow
1 handful Chinese cabbage
3 broccoli florets
½ cup seedless grapes
1 kiwi fruit
½-in ginger root, peeled
1 cup filtered alkaline water or coconut water

NUTRITIONAL NUGGET
All the green vegetables included in these wonderful smoothies are rich in alkaline ingredients. Chlorophyll (the green pigment) cleanses and hydrates the intestines. Magnesium ensures that there's proper peristalsis in the gut and balanced heart function. They're also rich in highly absorbable iron.

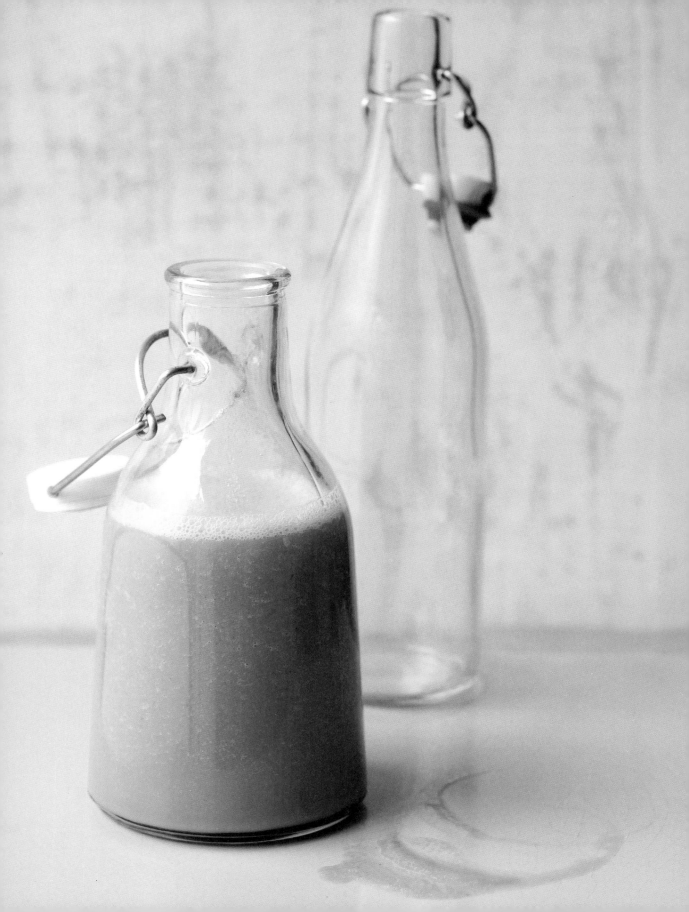

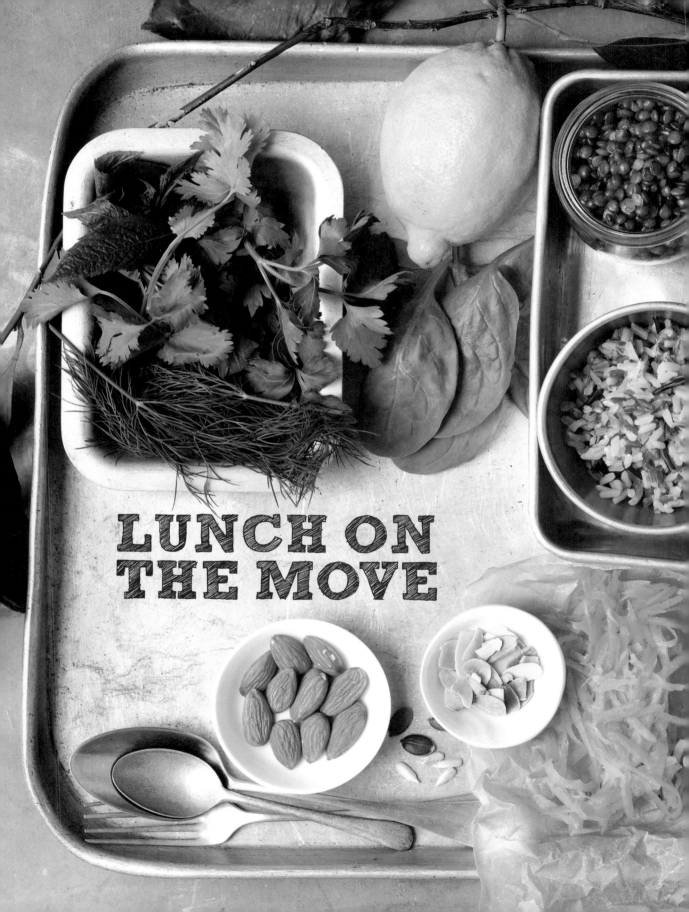

LUNCH ON THE MOVE

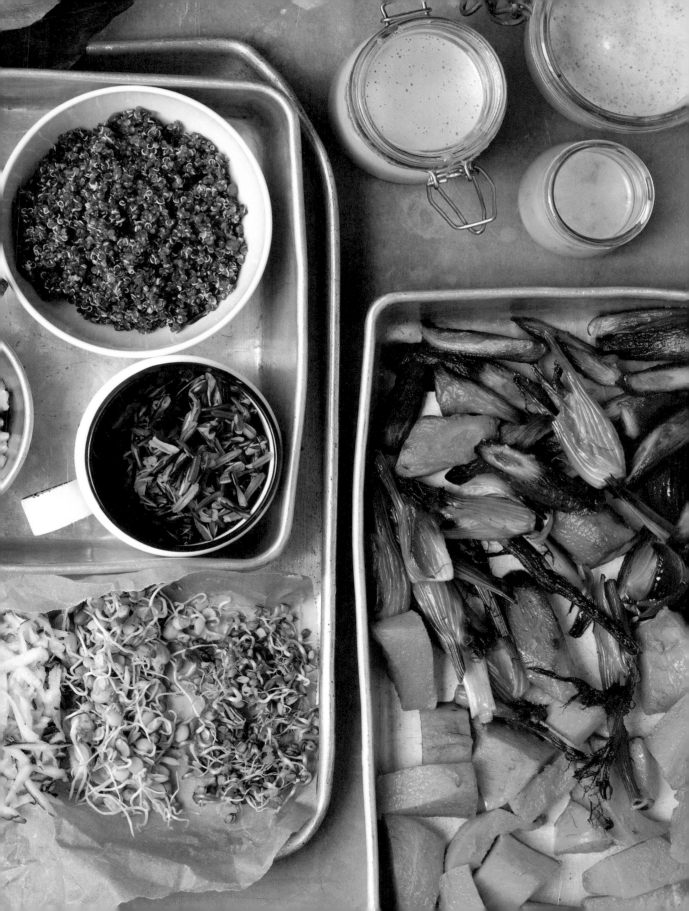

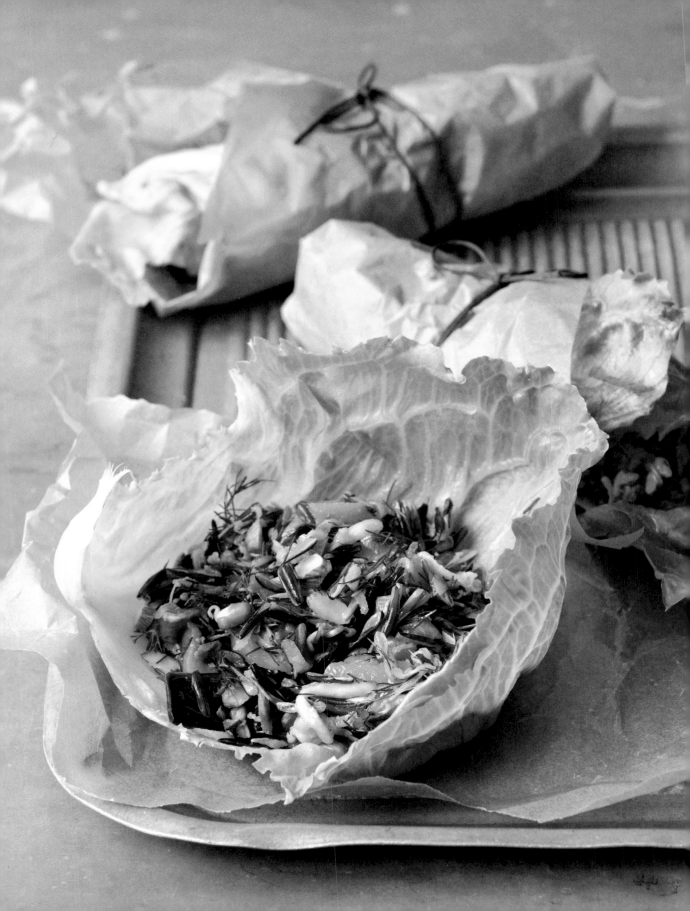

SALAD WRAPS

The idea behind these wraps is to show you different combinations from recipes throughout the book either as a salad or as a wrap without the bread. But it's all about preparation; if you have already made some of the recipes below then you can use any leftovers to throw together a quick and easy on-the-go lunch.

Throughout the book there are loads of side dishes, dressings, and salads that can all become wonderfully tasty combinations. Here are a few to get you started, but have a go and be creative...it's time to put on your chef's hat.

Step 1

Start with a legume or a grain.
(Cook according to package instructions.)
Puy lentils
Red rice
Quinoa
Brown rice

Step 2

Add a cooked or roasted vegetable.
Rainbow Salad with Roasted Vegetables,
   see page 205
Masala Roasted Root Vegetables, see page 131
Baked Spiced Eggplant, see page 78
Roasted Rainbow Carrots, see page 110
Roasted butternut squash, from Peach and
   Butternut Salad, see page 202

Step 3

Add something raw.
Grated carrot
Grated zucchini
Kale massaged with a little lemon juice
Chopped cabbage
Spinach

Step 4

Add chopped herbs.
Flat-leaf parsley
Cilantro
Chervil
Dill

Step 5

Add a dressing or a dip (choose from those on page 82).

Step 6

Sprinkle with nuts or seeds; you could add tofu, too, if you like.

Step 7

Mix it all together.
Either pile your mix on top of a bed of fresh leaves or use as a filling for a wrap made of lightly steamed chard leaves or large iceberg lettuce leaves.

TASH'S TIPS
Three of my favorite combinations are:
1 Red rice, eggplant with cinnamon, grated carrot, flat-leaf parsley with Tahini Dressing (see page 82), and pumpkin seeds.
2 Puy lentils, roasted butternut squash, kale, dill, smoked tofu, and minty yogurt dressing.
3 Quinoa, roasted rainbow carrots, spinach, chervil, sesame seeds, and sweet chili sauce.

PUY LENTIL, BROWN RICE, AND SWEET POTATO SALAD

This dish tastes equally fabulous warm or cold. If you are eating it warm, follow the method below. However, if you fancy taking it to lunch at work or on a picnic then simply make each part of the recipe individually, put the dressing in a little pot or jar, and then just mix together when and where you want to eat it.

serves 4

1 cup brown basmati rice

¾ cup Puy lentils

1 piece kombu seaweed

2 large sweet potatoes (about 15 oz), peeled and cut into ¾-in cubes

3 tbsp sunflower oil

a pinch of ground coriander

⅓ cup frozen edamame, defrosted

⅓ cup dill, chopped

1 scallion, finely sliced at an angle

1 tbsp raw cashew nuts (optional), halved or whole, to garnish

flat-leaf parsley, to garnish

For the dressing:

⅓ cup flat-leaf parsley, chopped

⅓ cup sesame oil

1 lemon

a pinch of Himalayan pink salt

For the tamari-roasted seed topping:

⅓ cup raw pumpkin seeds

2 tbsp tamari

Preheat the oven to 350°F.

Cook the brown rice and Puy lentils according to the package instructions; brown rice will take 40 minutes while Puy lentils take a bit less, more like 25 minutes. When cooking the lentils add a piece of kombu seaweed (see also page 211) to help break down the complex sugars that can cause bloating and gas.

When the brown rice is halfway through its cooking time, put the sweet potatoes onto a baking sheet, drizzle with the sunflower oil, and sprinkle with ground coriander. Bake in a preheated oven for 20 minutes.

Next, mix the pumpkin seeds with the tamari to get a good coating and put onto a baking sheet. Roast in the preheated oven for 10 minutes. Remove from the oven and let cool, then use as the garnish.

Put all the ingredients for the dressing into a blender and whiz up for around 30 seconds.

Put the cooked rice and lentils, edamame, dill, roasted sweet potato, and scallion into a large bowl with half of the dressing and mix thoroughly.

To serve, divide the mixture between four plates and drizzle the remaining dressing over the top. Garnish with cashew nuts, if using, tamari-roasted seeds, and parsley.

NUTRITIONAL NUGGET

Edamame are a great source of insoluble fiber, bone-building minerals, and a complete range of amino acids. As an unprocessed source of soy, you can't get better than eating the beans themselves— and do try to source organic.

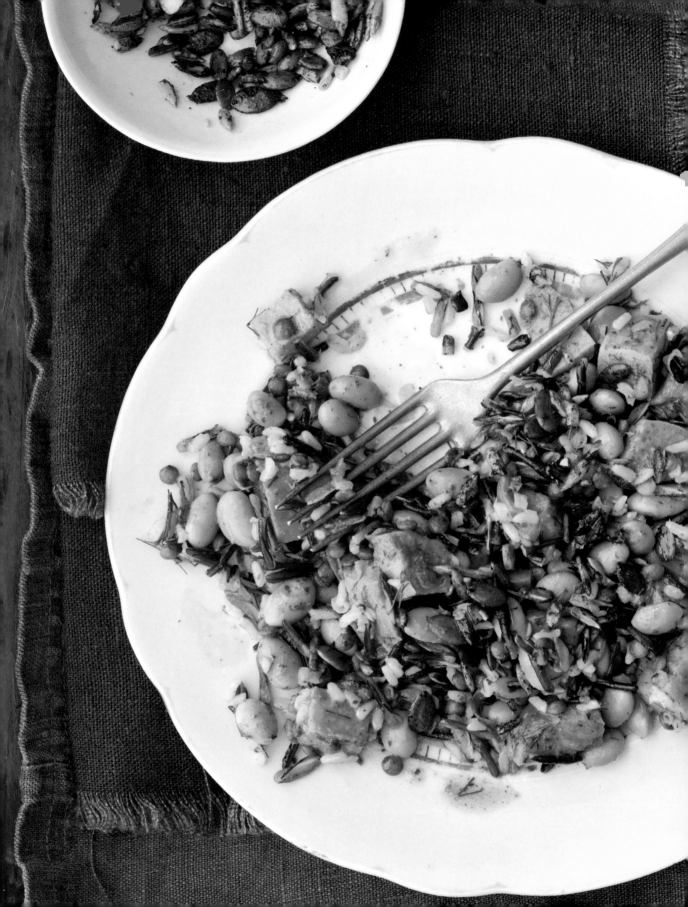

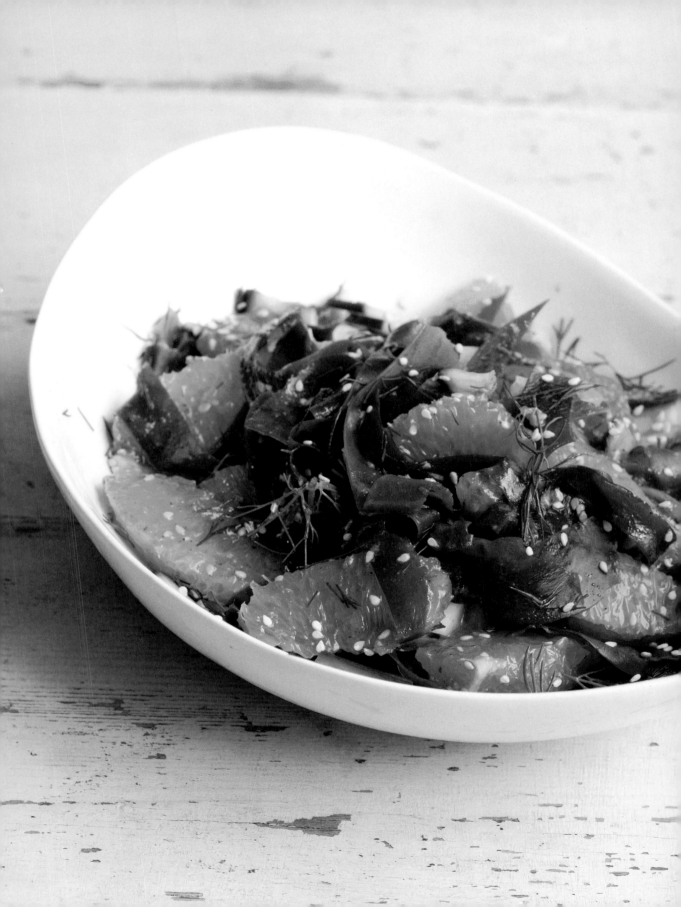

CITRUS SEAWEED SALAD

*Just throw all of the ingredients into a tub and add
the dressing when you're ready to eat—this is a
fantastic "make and dash" dish.*

serves 2 as a side dish

1¼ oz wakame seaweed

1 grapefruit, peeled and segmented

1 orange, peeled and segmented

2-in cucumber, chopped into thin cubes

1 scallion, finely sliced at an angle

½ cup dill, chopped

1 tbsp sesame seeds

2 tbsp Asian Dressing (see page 82)

Soak the seaweed in warm water for 15 minutes.
Drain, then cut the stalks off and slice the rest into
½-inch wide strips.

Combine all of the ingredients and toss with your
hands until integrated.

TASH'S TIPS
If you are in need of a more substantial
meal, try adding cooked brown rice,
which goes perfectly with this salad.

NUTRITIONAL NUGGET
Seaweeds are one of the most
alkaline foods, providing not only the
broadest range of amino acids but
also a rich supply of vitamin C,
calcium, and iron.

RAW GREEN CURRY WITH ZUCCHINI "NOODLES"

This is one of the most beautiful salads but is curious, too—it's so light but filling at the same time. The spiralized noodles are such a great touch, especially if you are trying to stay away from carbs. Why not use them instead of pasta with A Great Tomato Sauce (see page 221) if you're trying to steer clear of wheat? You may never look back.

serves 4 to 5

For the sauce:
⅓ cup dried or fresh curry leaves
1 cup raw cashew nuts, soaked for 30 minutes
    and drained
½ cup water
juice of ½ lime
½ cup cilantro, chopped
generous ¾ cup coconut milk
1 tsp each of ground cumin, ground ginger,
    dried lemongrass, fresh chili (chopped),
    garlic (chopped), ginger root (grated),
    ground coriander

For the zucchini "noodles":
5 zucchini
1 cup bean sprouts
1½ cups snow peas
2 red bell peppers, sliced
⅓ cup sugar snap peas, finely sliced
7 oz baby corn, sliced
raw cashew nuts, to garnish

Put all the sauce ingredients in a blender and whiz until smooth. Set aside.

Using a spiralizer (see also page 206), spiralize the zucchini, and then mix all the sauce over these "noodles" and add in the chopped vegetables. Pack into containers and refrigerate until ready to serve or eat. (If you prefer you can make the sauce a day or so ahead and mix with spiralized noodles just before serving.)

Garnish with a sprinkle of cashews just before eating.

TASH'S TIPS
If you don't have a high-speed blender, be sure to soak the cashews for a few hours, then they'll blend a lot easier; no one wants a lumpy sauce.

NUTRITIONAL NUGGET
Bean sprouts are a "living" food— that ensures all the protein therein is at its highest available level. Adding these to any dish completes the protein requirement for a meal, as well as having the satisfying crunchiness of such fresh foods.

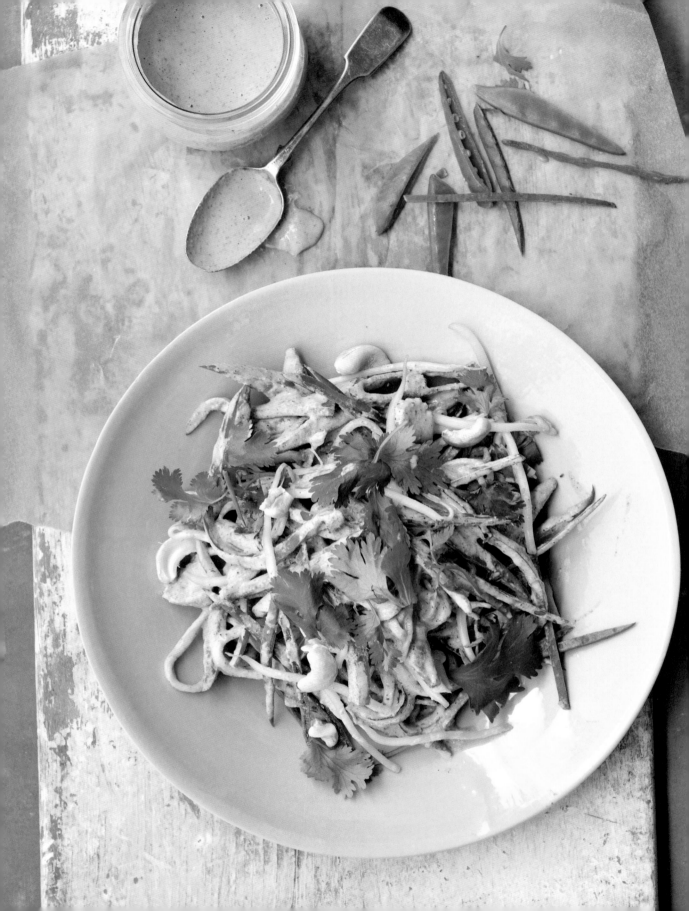

QUINOA, LEMON KALE, AND SESAME BEET SALAD

Bee pollen is a delicious sweet option on this salad, if you don't have it you can always leave it out, but I like the way it adds a delightful crunch. This salad can be made in advance and taken to work, just keep the dry ingredients separate from the wet ones and combine when you want to eat.

serves 4

3 large beets, peeled and chopped into half
   moon slices

3 tbsp sunflower oil

1 cup quinoa

1 tbsp bouillon powder

2 cloves garlic, crushed

1 small leek, finely sliced at an angle

juice of 1½ lemons

⅓ cup water

1½ cups kale, chopped

a pinch of Himalayan pink salt

½ cup purple sprouting broccoli tops, finely
   chopped

finely grated zest of 1 lemon

⅓ cup mint, chopped

⅓ cup flat-leaf parsley, chopped

¼ tbsp za'atar

½ tbsp mirin

1 tbsp sesame oil

1 tbsp brown rice vinegar

1 tsp bee pollen (optional; leave out to make it
   vegan), to garnish

Preheat the oven to 350°F.

Roast the beet for 45 minutes with 1 tablespoon of the sunflower oil.

Cook the quinoa as per the package instructions, including the bouillon powder, then set aside.

Heat the remaining sunflower oil in a pan until hot. Toss in the garlic and leeks and sauté over medium heat for 2 minutes. Add the juice of half a lemon and the measured water. Once the leeks have started to absorb some of the water, add the kale and stir. Next, add in the juice of another half a lemon along with a pinch of salt. Cook for 2 to 3 minutes until the kale is wilted and soft. Remove from the heat.

Assemble the ingredients by mixing the kale, leeks, and beets with the quinoa, then gently fold in the broccoli, lemon zest, and herbs.

Mix in the remaining lemon juice, za'atar, mirin, sesame oil, and brown rice vinegar. Finish off with a beautiful garnish of bee pollen, if using.

NUTRITIONAL NUGGET

Kale is the superfood of all dark green vegetables, with all the micronutrients in abundance—iron, manganese, magnesium, phosphorus, zinc, and vitamins C, E, and K make this potent strong-leafed vegetable number one on our nutrient-density list of alkaline foods.

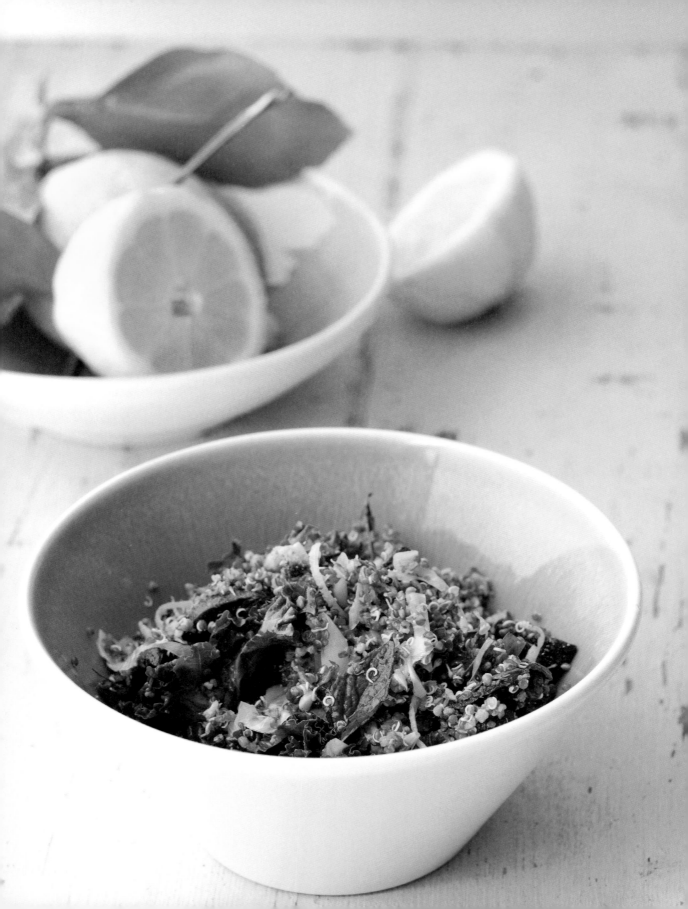

SUNDAY PREP

BAKED SPICED EGGPLANT

This dish has oh-so-many uses—it's a perfect side dish, a great addition to a salad, or drizzle with some Tahini Dressing (see page 82) and you have a fabulous dinner. It's definitely one to prepare in advance for the week ahead.

serves 4 as a side dish

1 eggplant

½ red onion, finely sliced

¼ tsp ground ginger

a pinch of Himalayan pink salt

¼ tsp caraway seeds or ground cinnamon

3 tbsp sunflower oil

Preheat the oven to 325°F. You'll need some parchment paper and an ovenproof dish.

First, you need to make a parchment parcel for the eggplant. Line the bottom of the ovenproof dish with parchment paper, leaving plenty all around the sides to be able to contain the eggplant and also make a lid of parchment to close the parcel.

Chop the eggplant into half-moon slices around 1¼-inches thick. Place in the bottom of the paper parcel followed by the onion, ground ginger, salt, and caraway seeds or cinnamon (whichever you're using). Drizzle over with the sunflower oil.

Cover with the parchment paper—your lid—to complete the parcel, and make sure the ends are all twisted and folded up so that no steam escapes.

Bake in a preheated oven for 45 minutes until soft and buttery to the touch. Remove from the oven and choose whichever way you'd like to eat this serving of deliciousness.

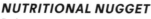

NUTRITIONAL NUGGET
Red onions are stronger than their white counterparts, and are a rich source of sulfur, to support optimal liver function and natural detoxification.

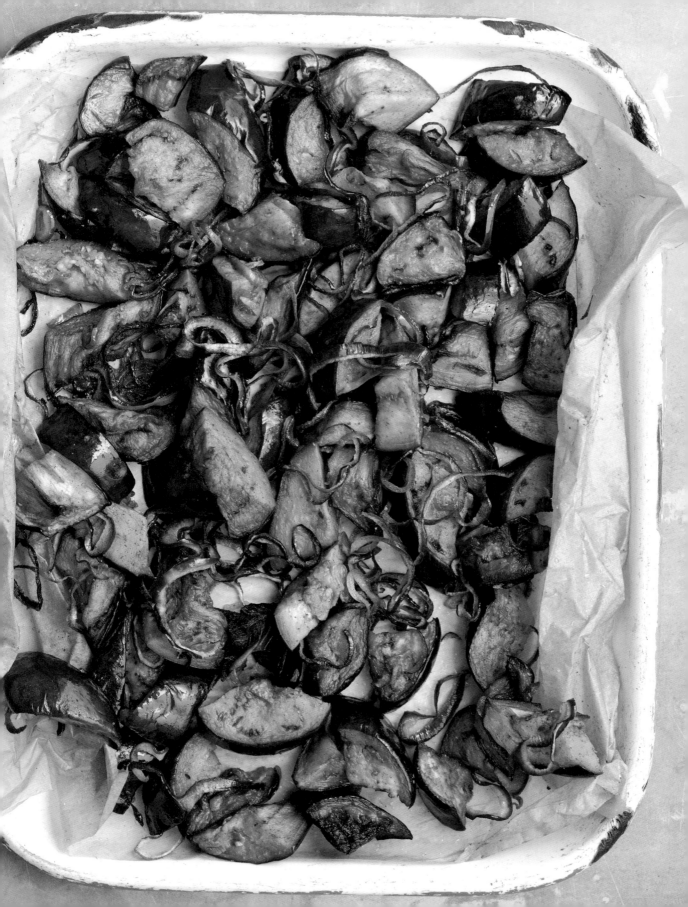

ASPARAGUS FRITTATA

Take advantage of asparagus when it's in season to make this frittata, which you can enjoy throughout the week. Whether you want to nibble on this for a snack or eat with a big green salad, it tastes divine.

serves 4

12–14 asparagus spears

8 eggs

3 scallions

1¼ oz dill

1¼ oz cilantro

a pinch of Himalayan pink salt

4 tsp sunflower oil or sunflower seed butter

1 tbsp raw sesame seeds

Preheat the oven to 325°F.

Trim the bottoms off the asparagus and then slice them lengthwise down the middle; if they're quite thick, you could cut each length in half again.

Bring a pan of water with 1 tablespoon of table salt to a rolling boil and put your asparagus in for 1 minute. Drain the asparagus and run under ice-cold water till cold.

Crack your eggs into a large mixing bowl and whisk. Thinly slice the scallions at a sharp angle, roughly chop the dill and cilantro, and add all of these to the egg mixture. Season with a pinch of Himalayan pink salt.

Heat the oil in a nonstick, heavy-bottom, ovenproof skillet over medium heat. Toss the sesame seeds into the skillet and as soon the seeds start changing color, to a golden brown, pour in the egg mixture.

Evenly arrange the asparagus on top of the egg mixture in the skillet and then put the skillet into the oven for 15 minutes, or until the egg is firm.

Slice in the skillet, remove each slice, and serve with a large side salad and sprouts tossed in our Perfect Salad Dressing (see page 82).

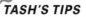

TASH'S TIPS

The only time I would use table salt is to blanch the asparagus. This is because, when blanching green veggies, if you boil them in very salty water, the salt acts as a barrier to osmosis, not allowing any nutrients to leave the veggies, and also makes them extremely green by drawing out the chlorophyll in them—you don't have to worry, though, as the salt does not penetrate the vegetable so the asparagus is not salty.

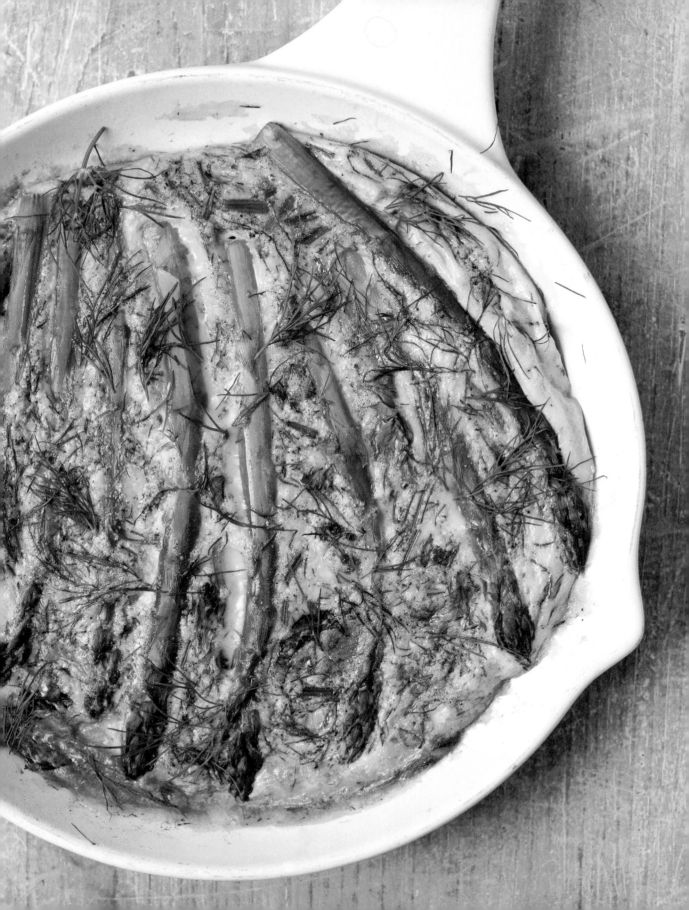

DRESSINGS AND MARINADES

Place all the ingredients for the dressings or marinades in a blender and blend well.
I like to make up a batch (so there's always some to drizzle) and keep it in a glass jar.

Asian Dressing or Marinade

♥ ♥ ♥

1 tsp lemongrass
1 tsp chili, finely chopped
⅛ tsp black onion seed
1 lime leaf
2 tbsp olive oil
1 tbsp tamari
½ tsp coconut palm sugar
1 slice ginger root
1 sprig of cilantro, chopped
1 tbsp sesame oil
1 tbsp water
½ clove garlic

Tahini Dressing

♥ ♥ ♥

2 tbsp sesame seed paste
¼ clove garlic
1 tbsp tamari
2 tbsp sesame oil
2 tbsp water
1 sprig of cilantro, chopped

Perfect Salad Dressing

♥ ♥ ♥

1 tsp Dijon mustard
1 tbsp agave syrup
3 tbsp olive oil
½ clove garlic
2 tbsp lemon juice
1 tbsp fresh rosemary
little pinch of Himalayan pink salt

Nice and Spicy Marinade

♥ ♥ ♥ ♥

2 tbsp lime juice
½ tsp smoked paprika
¼ tsp salt
⅛ tsp black pepper
6 tbsp olive oil
3 mint leaves, chopped

Herby Yogurt Dressing

♥ ♥

½ tsp cilantro, chopped
3 mint leaves, chopped
scant ½ cup dairy-free or
    goat's yogurt
½ clove garlic
⅛ tsp Himalayan pink salt
2 tbsp water

Minty Yogurt Dressing

♥ ♥

scant ¼ cup dairy-free or
    goat's yogurt
6 mint leaves, chopped
1 sprig of cilantro, chopped
¼ tsp smoked paprika
¼ clove garlic
1 tsp olive oil
a pinch of Himalayan pink salt

Sweet Chili Dipping Sauce

♥ ♥ ♥

2 tbsp brown rice syrup
1 tsp chili, finely chopped
¼ tsp ginger root, finely grated
¼ tsp garlic, finely chopped
¼ tsp lemongrass, finely chopped
1 tbsp lime juice
½ tsp cilantro, chopped

Simply mix all the ingredients
for the sauce together and serve.

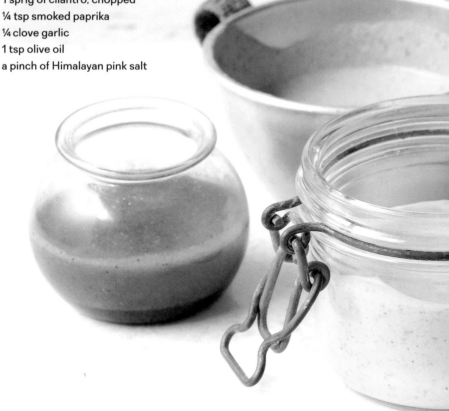

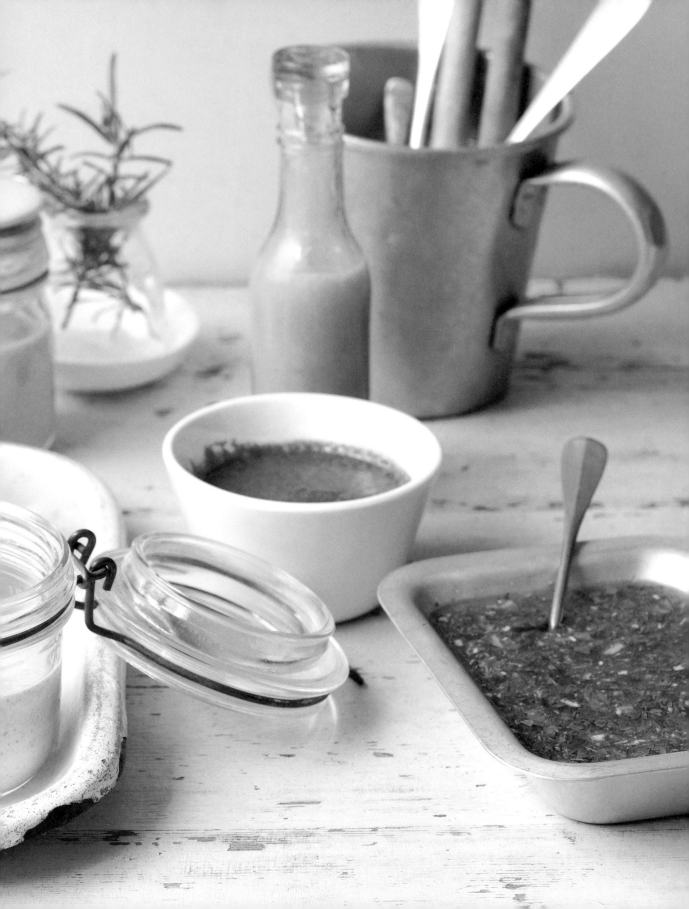

SNACKS

CHOCOLATE KALE CHIPS

These are an indulgent treat with an added element of green goodness! If you don't have a dehydrator, you can do them in the oven as well, so don't despair. I love to take these chips to nibble on during a long flight or car journey.

makes 5 snack portions

5½ oz kale leaves

4 tbsp raw cacao powder

2 tbsp agave syrup

scant ¼ cup coconut oil, melted

a pinch of Himalayan pink salt

Preheat a dehydrator to 145.4°F. (Alternatively, put the oven on its lowest setting.)

Remove the kale leaves from their stalks and chop into 2-inch pieces.

In a high-speed blender, add the raw cacao powder, agave syrup, coconut oil, and salt, and blend until the mixture is smooth.

In a bowl, using your hands, coat the kale leaves in the rich mixture so that they are well covered but not dripping. If you cover them too thickly they will not dry out properly and will end up chewy instead of crunchy.

Place on a tray in the dehydrator for 14 hours. (Alternatively, put on a baking sheet in a preheated oven with the door ajar for 6 to 8 hours.)

Once dehydrated, the kale chips keep for a week in an airtight container, though they never last that long in my house!

NUTRITIONAL NUGGET
The combination of kale and cacao packs a veritable immune-supporting punch with the abundance of zinc, vitamin C, iron, and selenium.

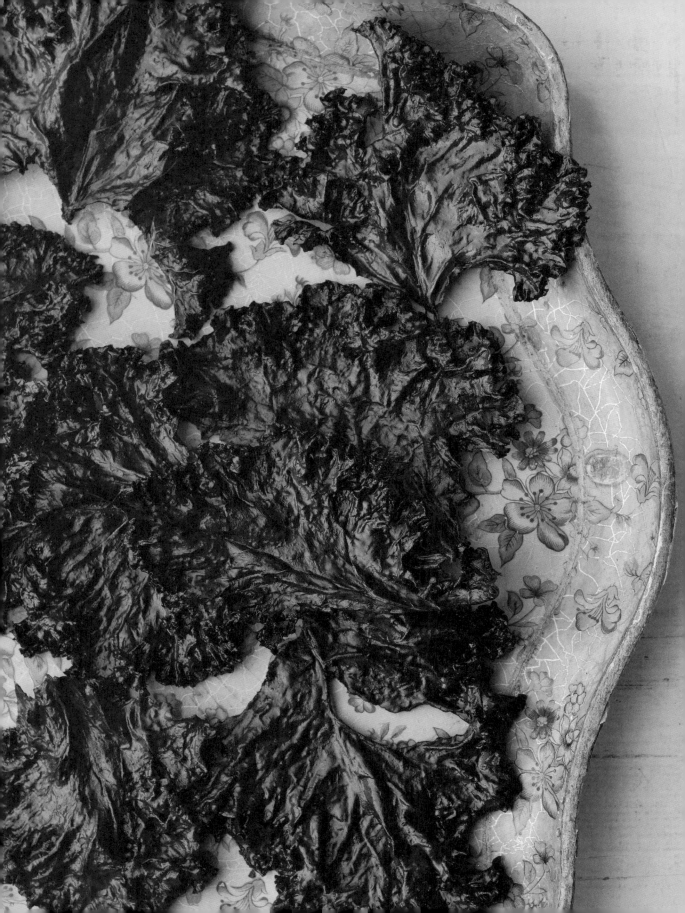

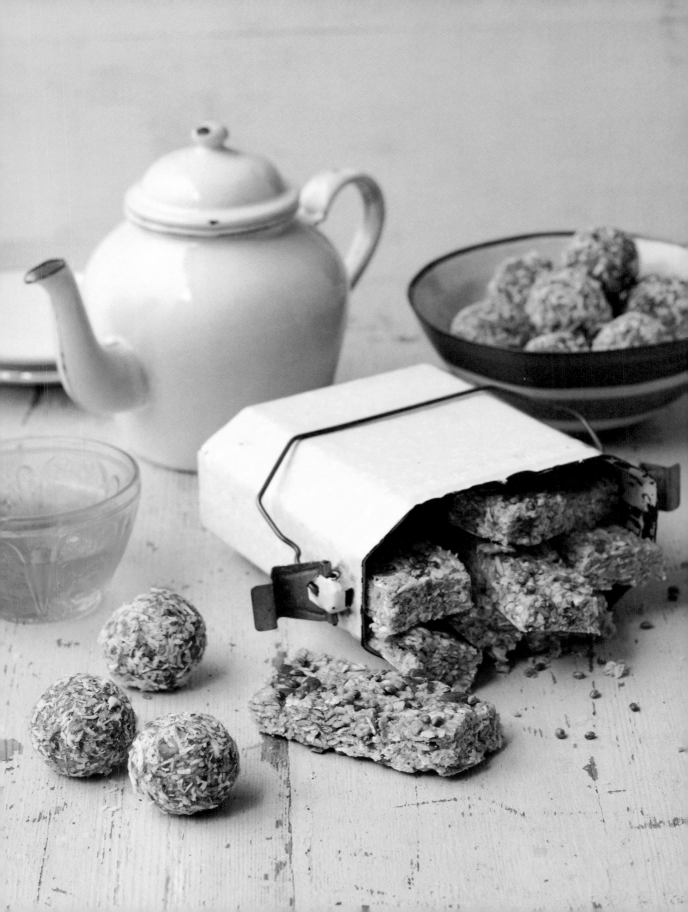

RAW HEMP GRANOLA BARS

These super-tasty and incredibly filling snacks are quick and easy to make and are all-round pleasers; kids love them, too. I eat them as an on-the-go breakfast or as an afternoon snack.

makes 12

2 cups dates, pitted

1 cup warm water

½ cup coconut oil, melted

1 tbsp vanilla extract

5¾ cups jumbo rolled oats

generous 1 cup dry unsweetened coconut

⅔ cup raw sunflower seeds

generous ¾ cup raw pumpkin seeds

⅓ cup raw hemp seeds

Line a baking sheet with parchment paper and set aside. Soak the dates in the warm water for 20 minutes. Then whiz in a high-speed blender with the water to make a smooth paste.

Melt the coconut oil in a heatproof bowl over a pan of simmering water or in a bain marie. Pour the oil into the blender along with the vanilla extract. Blend until smooth.

Put the oats, dry unsweetened coconut, sunflower seeds, and pumpkin seeds into a bowl, stir to mix, and then divide the mixture in half. Pulse half the mixture in a food processor, just roughly, so you maintain some texture.

Add the pulsed mixture back into the bowl of the "whole" mixture. Then pour the contents of the blender into the bowl and mix thoroughly so no dry ingredients remain. Pour the mixture onto the prepared baking sheet and pat down, so that it forms an even slab. Then scatter the hemp seeds over the top and press them into the slab. Refrigerate for 2 hours to set.

Remove from the refrigerator, cut into squares or rectangles, and enjoy; these keep for a week in an airtight container in the refrigerator.

SPIRULINA PROTEIN BALLS

These delicious balls of goodness are a perfect afternoon snack to keep energy levels and powers of concentration high—ideal for a post-workout snack. They're great for kids, too!

makes around 15 balls

7 dried figs

scant ¼ cup water

juice of 2 oranges (the zest is used too, so zest before juicing)

1 cup raw cashew nuts

scant 1 cup dry unsweetened coconut

¼ cup chia seeds

¼ cup raw pumpkin seeds

finely grated zest of 2 oranges

4 tbsp spirulina

½ cup coconut oil, melted

Blitz the figs in a blender with the water and orange juice to make a thick paste.

Pulse all the nuts, seeds, and orange zest in a food processor until you have a rough texture, then add the spirulina and half the melted coconut oil and pulse together until well mixed. Then add the remaining half of the oil along with the fig paste and mix again.

Take a small amount of mixture and roll into ping-pong-sized balls and put into the refrigerator to set for 20 to 30 minutes. These balls keep in an airtight container in the refrigerator for a week.

SUNDRIED TOMATO PESTO

Transport yourself to an Italian vacation with the colors and tastes of this simple pesto. It transforms the simplest of dishes from gluten-free pasta to grains, and it even works well as a dip.

makes around 2 cups

2 cups raw cashew nuts

4 oz sundried tomatoes, drained of oil

Simply blend both ingredients together or whiz in a food processor. There should be enough residual oil on the tomatoes to blend smoothly, but if not, add a little oil from the jar until the desired pesto consistency is reached.

SUNFLOWER SEED PASTE

Delicious and nutritious, this is brain food at its best! And it's quick to make, too. Whether you use it in a salad, spread it on a gluten-free cracker or on a slice of our Quinoa Bread (see page 95), you'll soon become a convert to this super-spread.

makes around ¾ cup

½ cup raw sunflower seeds

1 cup water

1 sundried tomato

juice of ¼ lemon

a pinch of Himalayan pink salt

1 tbsp olive oil

½ tsp finely chopped chili

⅓ cup mint, finely chopped

Soak the sunflower seeds in the measured water for two hours and drain. Then blend all the ingredients up to and including the olive oil together, then add the chili and mint to finish off.

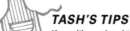

TASH'S TIPS

If you like a chunkier texture, set half the sunflower seeds aside and roughly blend them after you have already made the paste, then stir in to create some chunky bits throughout.

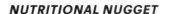

NUTRITIONAL NUGGET

Sunflower seeds are rich in selenium, zinc, and essential fatty acids, rendering them one of the smallest nutrient-dense foods we have available to us in the kitchen. Made into a paste, they provide a high-protein snack for any time of the day.

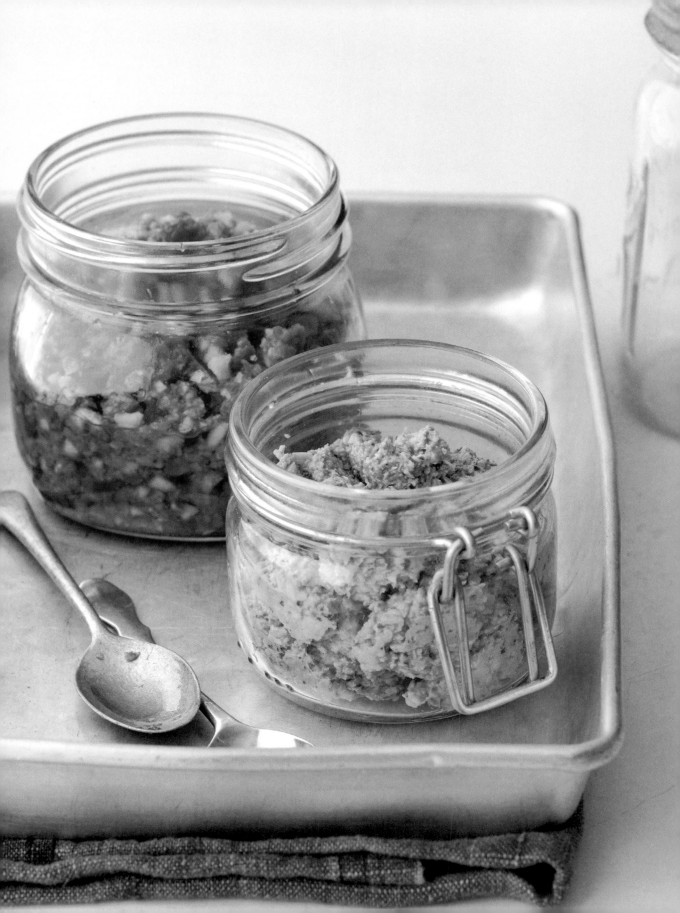

LAZY TIMES

I live for weekends and holidays—I love nothing more than to relax with friends and family, coming together with delicious, hearty food. In this section, you'll find everything you'd want from an indulgent lazy time, but made healthy! I hope you enjoy these cozy recipes as much as I do.

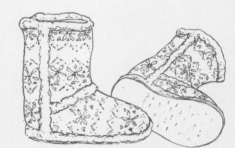

BREAKFAST IN BED

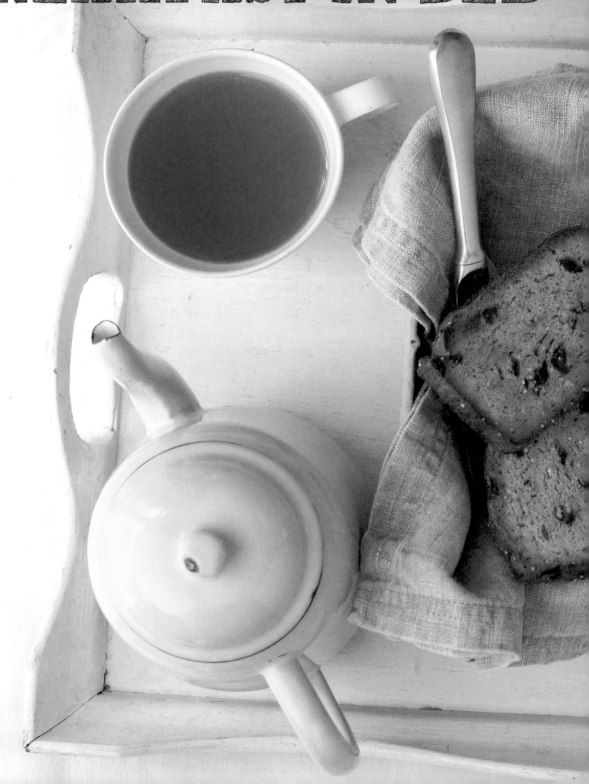

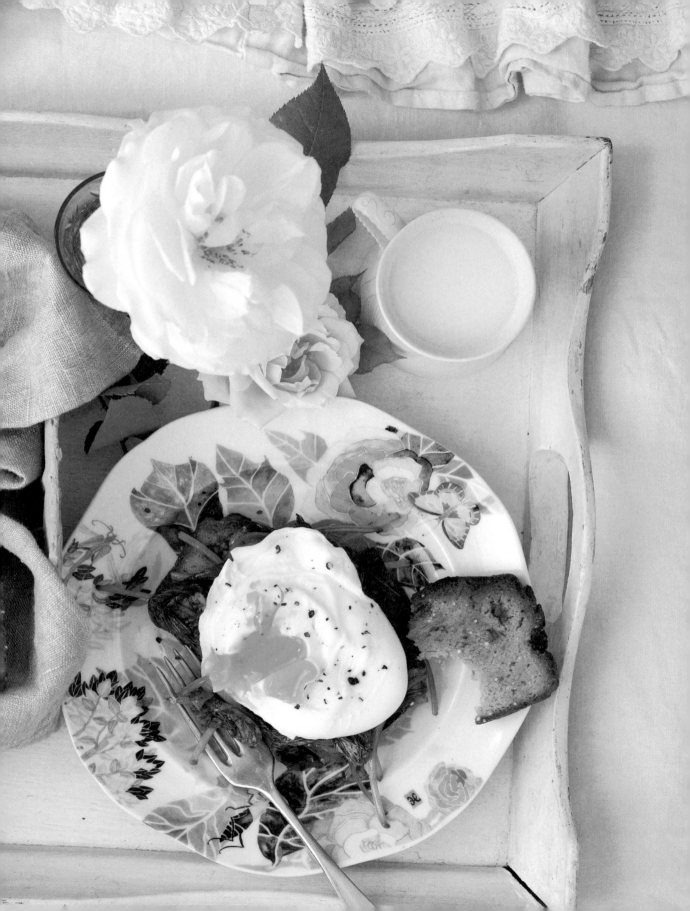

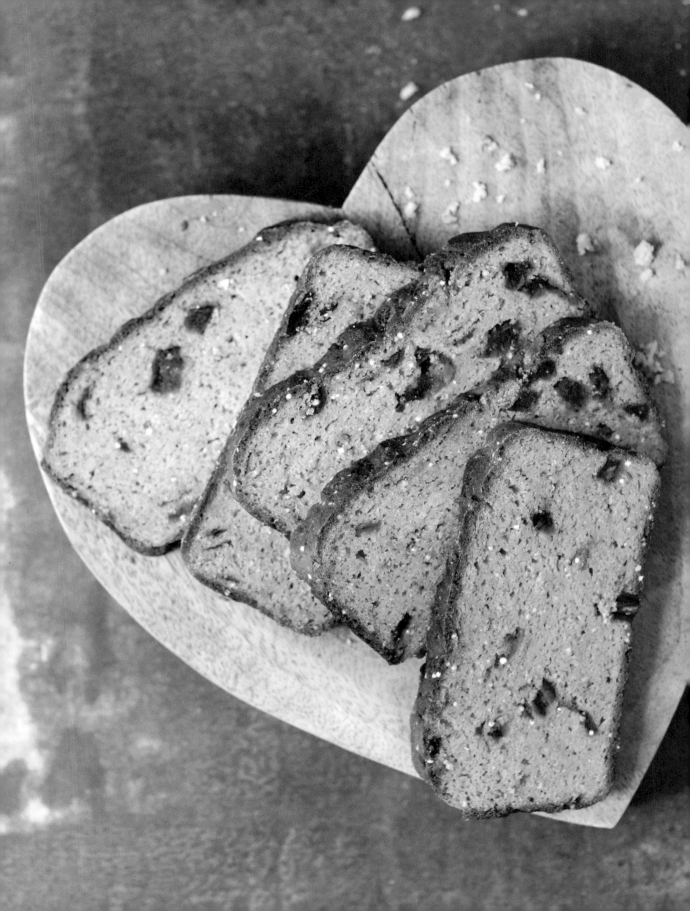

POACHED EGG AND SPINACH ON QUINOA TOAST

You'll find as long as you have some quinoa bread made, this dish works equally well for an indulgent weekend breakfast and for a "before work" quicky.

serves 1

1 tbsp sunflower oil

½ clove garlic, grated or crushed

1 egg

1 slice quinoa bread

1¼ oz washed baby spinach leaves

olive oil, for drizzling

cracked pepper

Fill a skillet with water to 1 inch from the top and bring to a boil.

At the same time, heat the sunflower oil in another skillet with the garlic and sauté for 1 minute.

When the water-filled skillet is at a rolling boil, turn it down to a simmer and crack the egg very carefully into the simmering water. Poach for 3 minutes (use a timer), making sure that the water completely covers the egg; if necessary, spoon cooking water over the egg while it cooks.

Meanwhile, pop the bread into the toaster or under the broiler.

When the garlic has softened in the other skillet, add the spinach and let it wilt for 30 to 60 seconds.

Place your toast onto a plate and pile the spinach on top. Carefully remove the egg from the water with a slotted spoon and place on the spinach. Drizzle with a little olive oil and cracked pepper.

Quinoa bread

makes 1 loaf

2½ tsp or 1 packet fast-action dried yeast

½ cup warm water

1 tbsp agave syrup

¾ cup brown rice flour

¾ cup almond flour

½ cup quinoa flour

½ cup buckwheat flour

2 tbsp coconut flour (you can use more almond
   flour instead as this is expensive)

⅓ cup quinoa flakes, plus extra for sprinkling

1 tsp xanthan gum

1 tsp fine sea salt

scant ¼ cup olive oil

3 eggs, beaten

⅓ – ½ cup warm water

scant ½ cup pitted dates, chopped

First, activate the yeast. Sprinkle the dried yeast into ½ cup warm water and stir in the agave syrup. Set aside for 15 minutes.

In a large bowl, whisk together the flours, quinoa flakes, xanthan gum, and sea salt. Make a well in the center and pour in the yeast mixture. Then add the olive oil and eggs. Start beating it together. As you beat, dribble in some warm water a tablespoon at a time, until the batter is smooth, akin to a thick muffin batter. You'll need around ⅓ – ½ cup of warm water. When fully mixed, add in the chopped dates and mix through.

Grease a 9-inch loaf pan and scoop the bread dough into the prepared pan, smooth out the top, and sprinkle with quinoa flakes.

Allow the dough to rest and rise in a warm place for 50 minutes. After 30 minutes preheat the oven to 350°F.

Bake in a preheated oven for 55 to 60 minutes, until crusty and browned. Remove from the oven, let cool slightly, and transfer to a wire rack to cool.

MY FAVORITE GRANOLA

*What better way to start your day than with one
of my favorite breakfasts? Just make a big batch
of this granola when you have the time and grab a
bowl before work. No excuses to skip breakfast now!*

makes 1 lb 11¾ oz (a large Mason jar)

5¾ cups gluten-free jumbo oats

4 tbsp sunflower oil

scant ½ cup agave syrup

1 tsp ground cinnamon

scant ¼ cup raw sesame seeds

scant ½ cup raw pumpkin seeds

⅓ cup raw sunflower seeds

½ cup raw whole almonds

⅔ cup dried apricots, chopped

Preheat the oven to 300°F, and line a baking sheet
with parchment paper.

Put the oats into a large bowl and coat them with
the sunflower oil, agave syrup, cinnamon, and
sesame seeds.

Scatter the oats evenly over the baking sheet and
bake in the preheated oven. After 10 minutes they
should be golden on top—take them out of the oven
and stir them around so that all the oats become
golden. Return to the oven for 5 minutes.

Once all the oats are nice and golden, scatter the
seeds and nuts (I like them whole but you could
chop them if you prefer) over the top and bake for
another 8 minutes.

Remove from the oven and when cool mix in the
dried apricot and store in an airtight container.
This granola keeps for up to 3 months.

NUTRITIONAL NUGGET

Oats contain a specific type of fiber
known as beta-glucan, which has
been shown to lower blood
cholesterol levels, so they will keep
your heart and circulation healthy.

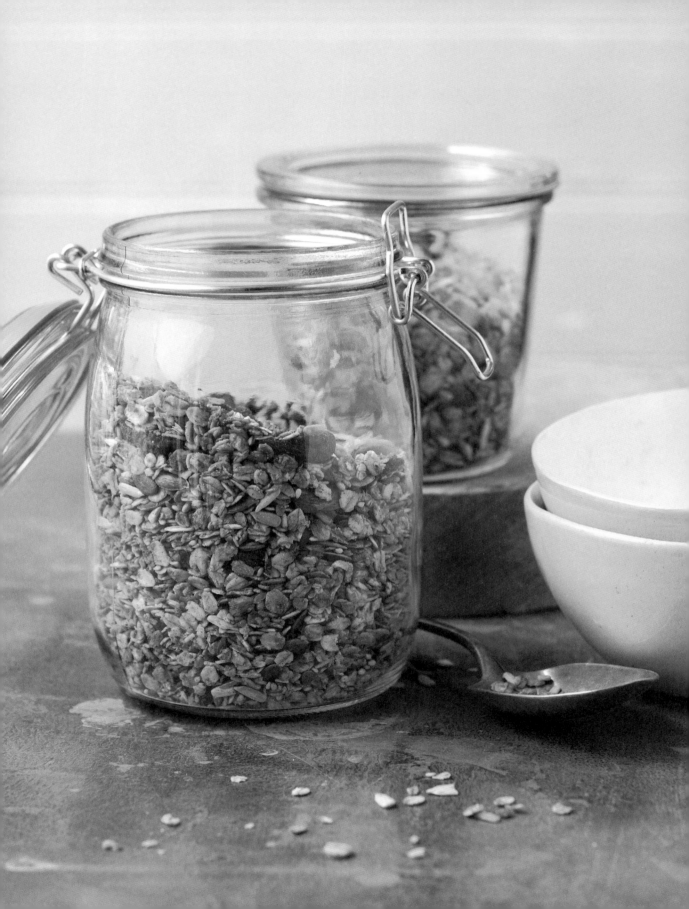

NUTTY BANANA MUFFINS

These little rays of breakfast sunshine are so enjoyable and too good to save just for the mornings—have one as an afternoon snack with one of our teas or tisanes on page 256.

makes 12

1 cup rice flour

¾ cup tapioca flour

½ cup buckwheat flour

2 tsp gluten-free baking powder

½ tsp baking soda

½ tsp Himalayan pink salt

1 tsp xanthan gum

½ tsp ground nutmeg

¼ cup sunflower oil

½ cup rice milk

scant 1 cup agave syrup

2 tsp vanilla extract

2 eggs

5 large, very ripe bananas, mashed

1¼ cups raw walnuts, chopped (keep 12 walnut halves aside for decorating the tops of the muffins)

Preheat the oven to 325°F and grease a 12-hole muffin pan really well and line with paper liners.

Sift together the dry ingredients (except the walnuts) and mix well with a fork.

Place all the liquids and the eggs in a food mixer, slowly add in the dry ingredients and mix until well combined. Stir in the mashed banana and the chopped walnuts and divide the batter between the paper liners. Pop the reserved walnut halves on the top of each muffin.

Bake in the preheated oven for 25 minutes, until cooked through and a skewer inserted into the center comes out clean.

Remove from the oven, let cool slightly in the pan, and transfer to a wire rack to cool.

TASH'S TIPS
Don't be tempted to eat these before they're completely cool as they could be a little soggy. Once cooled, though, they'll be wonderfully crumbly—just as a muffin should be.

NUTRITIONAL NUGGET
Buckwheat is rich in folic acid for balancing nerves, and rutin to support the tiny capillaries in legs, preventing thread veins.

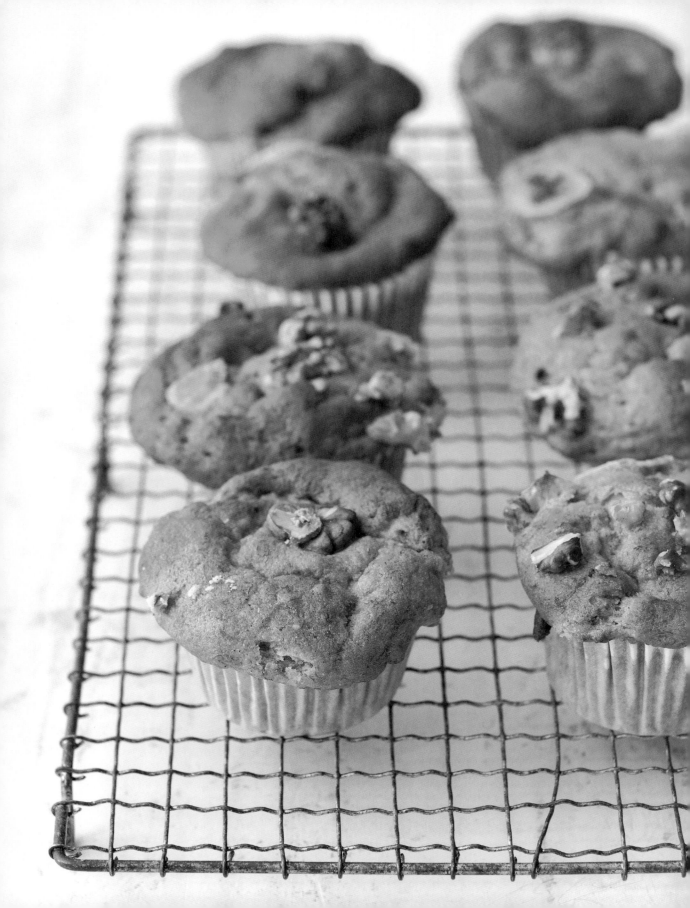

MOSES'S "NUTELLA"

I developed this grown-up version of the famous Nutella for my gorgeous nephew Moses as it's his favorite. Be warned, it is really delicious—I have been known to simply spoon it out of the jar when in need of a sweet fix.

makes around 2 cups

1⅔ cups raw hazelnuts

4 tbsp raw cacao powder

4 tbsp brown rice syrup

5 tbsp hazelnut milk

Preheat the oven to 325°F, and line a baking sheet with parchment paper. Put the hazelnuts on the baking sheet and bake for 20 minutes.

Remove from the oven, wait until the nuts are cool, then roll between your hands to remove the skins.

Next, place the hazelnuts in water so they are covered and soak for 30 minutes. Drain the nuts and put them into a blender with the cacao, syrup, and nut milk. Blend until lovely and smooth.

Keep it in an airtight container—a jar works well, too—in the refrigerator and use within 7 to 10 days.

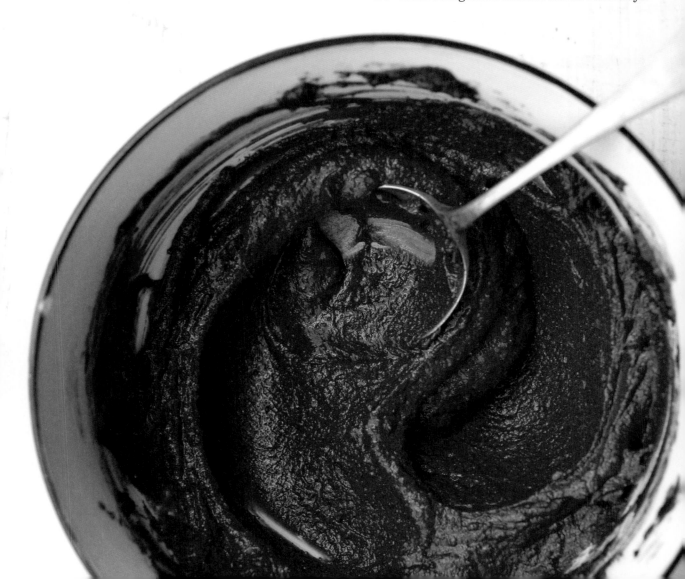

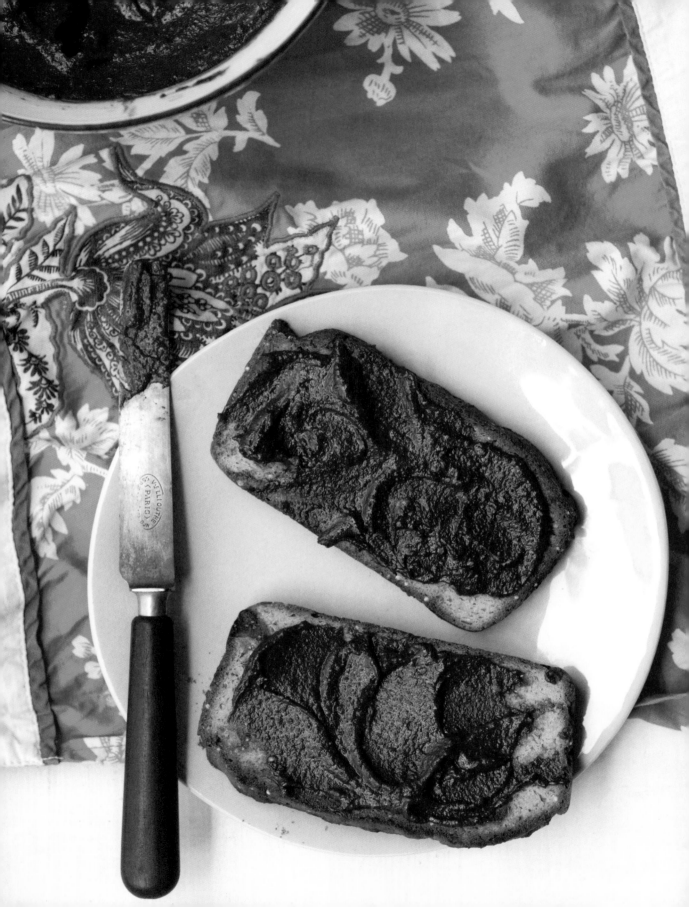

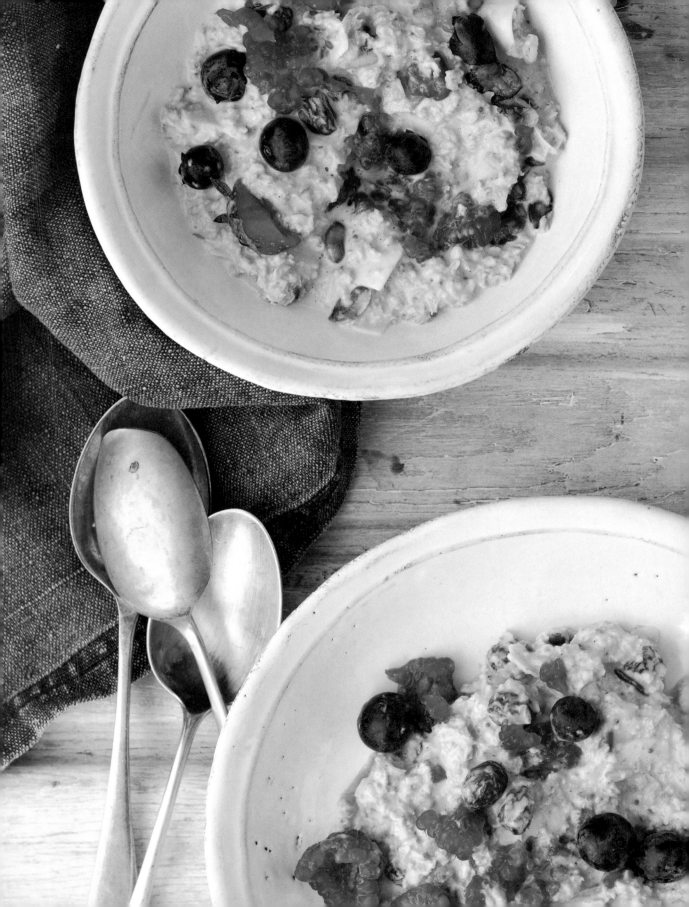

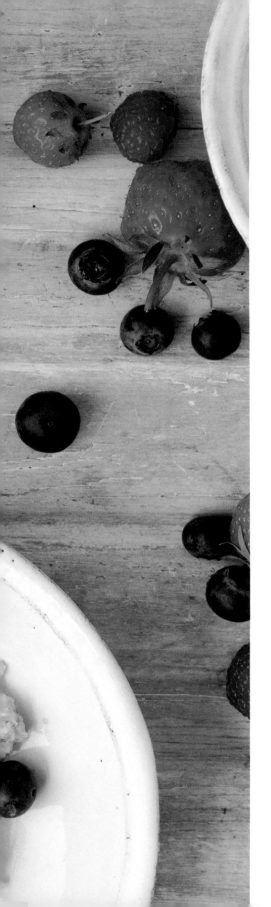

BIRCHER MUESLI

Make up a big batch of this breakfast goodie on a Sunday, or when you've got time, so you are set for a week's worth of breakfasts. Oats release their energy slowly, helping to stabilize your blood sugar levels throughout the day—and resulting in no cravings. Bonus! If you're making a batch for the week, I would double the quantities below.

serves 2

2¾ cups gluten-free rolled oats

½ tsp ground cinnamon

¼ cup coconut shavings

2 tbsp raw sunflower seeds

1 tbsp raw pumpkin seeds

½ cup raisins (or substitute chopped dried figs, dates, or apricots)

2 cups hot water

Mix all the dry ingredients together in a bowl. Simply add the water, give the mixture another good stir, and then leave to soak for a couple of hours or overnight in the refrigerator.

If it's really sticky after 2 hours, add a splash of extra water to loosen up the muesli; some oats are super-absorbent and others aren't, so it'll depend on the type you use.

Top with fresh fruit of your choice and enjoy.

NUTRITIONAL NUGGET

Cinnamon reduces inflammation ,as well as being naturally sweet, so reduces bloating—think of it as a flat tummy super-nutrient!

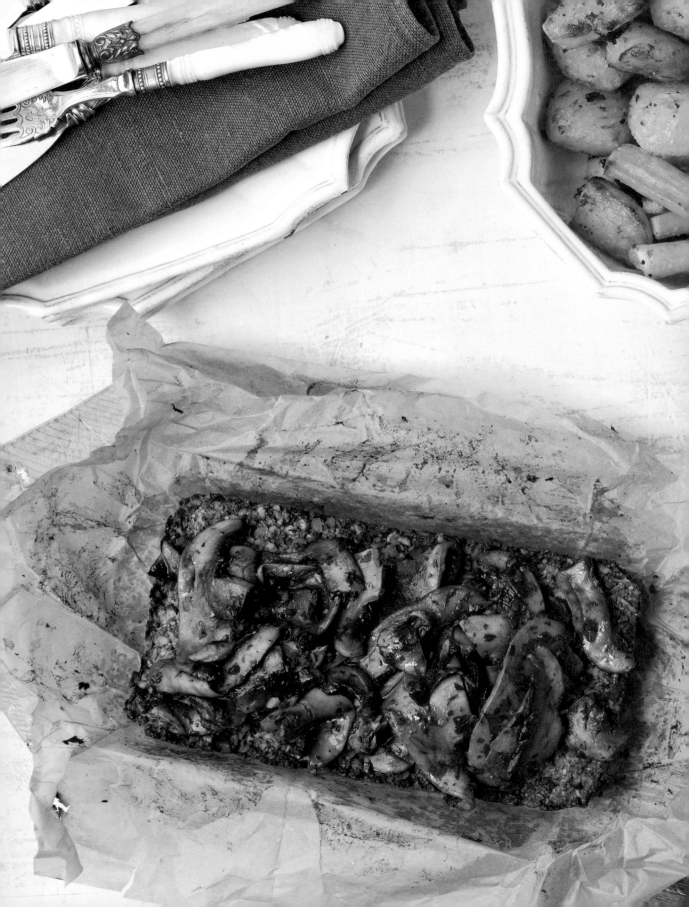

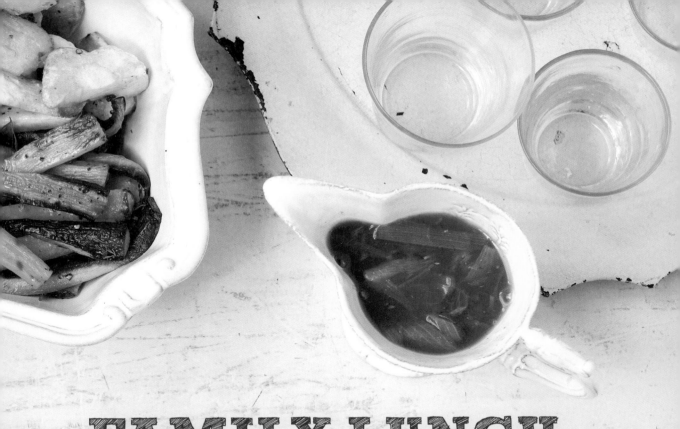

FAMILY LUNCH

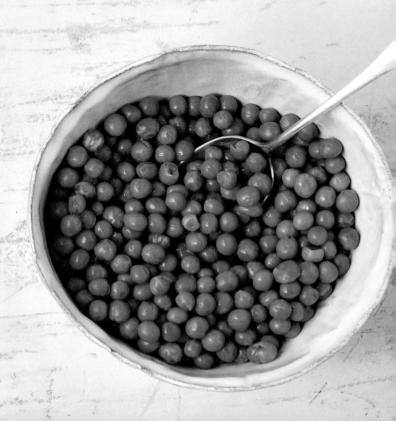

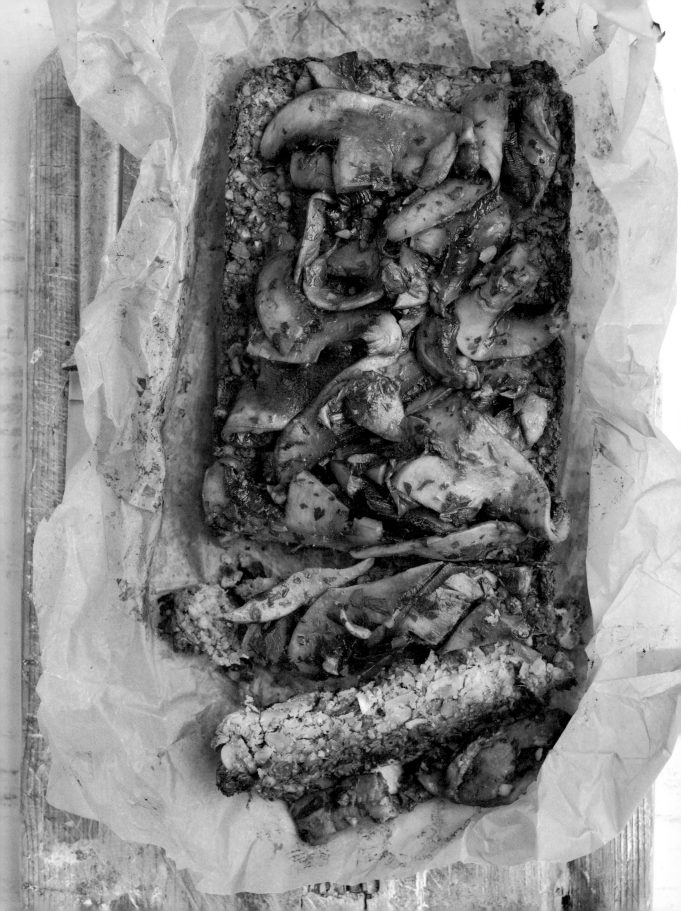

SAV'S NUT ROAST

My stepsister Savannah has always been an amazing cook and I love going round to her house for lunch, especially when she makes a nut roast. I've made a few little tweaks, though, so that it is now Honestly Healthy-friendly. She likes to add grated cheese to the top, so you could add some goat's cheese (¾ oz) for added indulgence; if you do, then add this five minutes before you take the roast out of the oven so it can melt beautifully on the top.

serves 4

⅔ cup raw walnuts
⅔ cup raw slivered almonds
scant ½ cup raw whole almonds
scant ½ cup raw pine nuts
⅔ cup raw brazil nuts
1 clove garlic
½ onion, chopped
1 large tomato, chopped
1 egg (optional, leave out if you want it vegan)
juice of 1 lemon
1 tbsp brown rice vinegar
⅛ tsp ground ginger
⅛ tsp ground allspice
¼ tsp ground coriander
¼ tsp umeboshi plum purée
⅓ cup flat-leaf parsley, chopped
3 tbsp vegan butter
3 large portobello mushrooms, chopped

Preheat the oven to 325°F, and line a 9-inch loaf pan with parchment paper.

Blitz the nuts, garlic, onion, tomato, and egg (if using) together in a food processor until roughly chopped then pour out into a bowl. Add the lemon juice, brown rice vinegar, ginger, allspice, ground coriander, plum purée, and half of the parsley and mix together thoroughly.

In a skillet, add the vegan butter, remaining parsley, and chopped mushrooms and gently sauté until the mushrooms are lovely and soft.

Tightly pack the nut mixture into the prepared pan and then pour the mushrooms over the top.

Bake in the preheated oven for 25 minutes.

Remove from the oven and serve straightaway with some peas, a dish of Roasted Veggies (see page 109), and a pitcher of gravy (see below).

Vegetarian Gravy

makes 3⅔ cups

1 large red onion or 2 small red onions
1 tbsp bouillon powder
2 sprigs rosemary
¼ lemon whole
3⅔ cups water
1 small carrot, quartered
1 small leek, chopped into large chunks
1 tbsp kuzu
1 tbsp water

Put all the ingredients, except the kuzu and measured water, in a medium-sized pan and cook over medium heat for 35–40 minutes, until the vegetables go soft and the liquid reduces.

In a small cup, dissolve the kuzu in 1 tablespoon of water and mix together until all the granules are absorbed and you have a milky water.

Add the kuzu mixture bit by bit into the gravy, stirring on the heat all the time; the kuzu will slowly thicken the gravy. Do add the kuzu slowly, otherwise it might overthicken suddenly; adjust the amount you put in based on whether you like a runny or thick gravy.

Serve with or without the cooked veggies (except the lemon) in the gravy. I like to keep them in, as they give the gravy a wonderful depth of flavor.

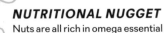

NUTRITIONAL NUGGET
Nuts are all rich in omega essential fats, which are great for the heart, and are packed with protein.

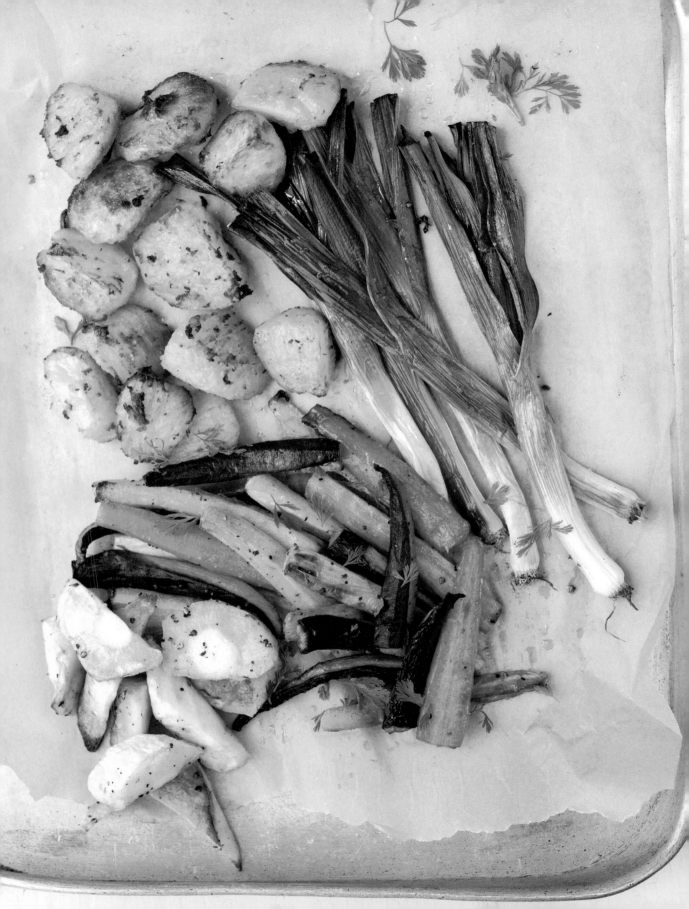

ROASTED VEGGIES

The easiest way to explain how to cook any selection of roast vegetables is according to their texture. Harder veggies need longer than softer ones—see my guide (on the right) for timings.

I like to roast my vegetables with a drizzle of sunflower oil. Experiment with different combinations of vegetables as well as spices and herbs; I do find the traditional rosemary or thyme with some whole garlic cloves is hard to beat.

Hard vegetables—take 40 to 50 minutes
Beet
Carrots
Parsnips
Turnips
Sweet potato
Celeriac
Jerusalem artichokes
Butternut squash or pumpkin

Softer vegetables—take 25 to 35 minutes
Fennel
Onions
Leeks
Eggplant
Garlic

Soft vegetables—take 15 to 25 minutes
Peppers
Zucchini
Asparagus
Tomatoes

LYRA'S PESTO

My gorgeous niece Lyra, when she was four years old, tried my pesto one day on holiday and said it was the best thing she had ever eaten. I promised I would put it in the new book and name it after her. She doesn't like cashews so I make it for her with pine nuts, but I prefer it with cashews—you can take your pick! But whichever you choose, you can be sure that both taste utterly delicious.

makes 1 cup

generous ¾ cup raw cashew nuts or raw pine nuts

3½ oz fresh basil leaves

scant ¼ cup olive oil

a pinch of Himalayan pink salt

½ clove garlic

2 oz hard sheep's cheese, such as Pecorino

juice of ½ lemon

Soak the cashews in water for 30 minutes, then drain. (There's no need to soak the pine nuts, if you're using those.)

Put the nuts along with the basil, olive oil, and salt in a high-speed blender and whiz until the nuts are broken down to a chunky paste.

Pour the contents out of the blender into a bowl and grate in the garlic and sheep's cheese (grate on the smallest possible setting, as if grating Parmesan), and then mix in the lemon juice.

Use straightaway or store in an airtight container in the refrigerator; this pesto lasts for a week. It's perfect to add to gluten-free pasta, enjoy as a dip, or use as a marinade.

ROASTED RAINBOW CARROTS

I find these work well with almost any dish, and the tamari gives it a wonderful saltiness so there's no need to season. They're also delicious piled onto a bed of leaves as a salad with our Tahini Dressing (see page 82) for an extra protein kick for a tasty and healthy lunch.

serves 4

1 lb 12¼ oz mixed colored carrots (you can use only orange carrots when rainbow carrots are not in season)

2 tbsp sesame oil

3 tbsp tamari

1 tbsp mixed sesame seeds

finely grated zest of 1 lemon

2 cups fresh chervil or flat-leaf parsley, roughly chopped

Preheat the oven to 325°F, and line a baking sheet with parchment paper.

Peel the carrots and cut them into rustic chunks at different angles. Put the carrots into a bowl with the sesame oil, tamari, and sesame seeds and toss well.

Place them on the prepared baking sheet and roast in a preheated oven for 25 minutes.

Remove from the oven. When they have cooled, mix the lemon zest and chervil or parsley through the carrots and serve straightaway.

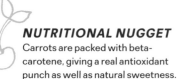

NUTRITIONAL NUGGET
Carrots are packed with beta-carotene, giving a real antioxidant punch as well as natural sweetness.

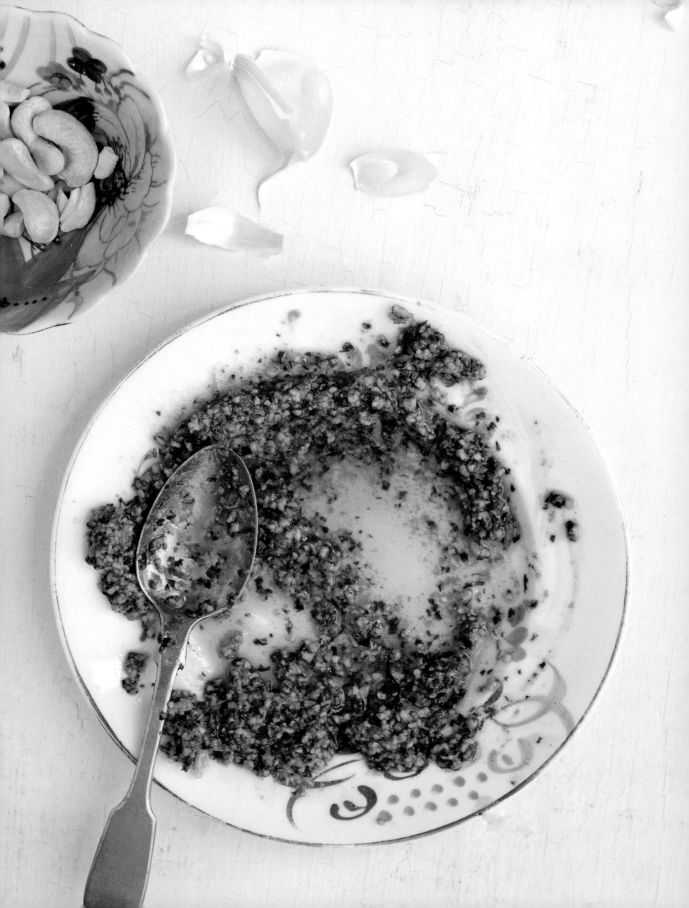

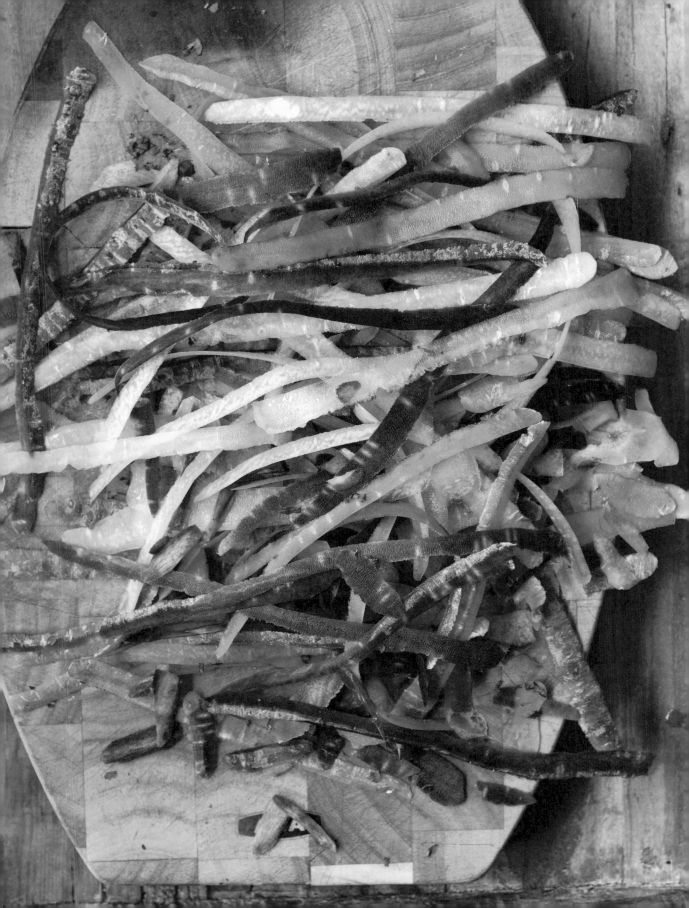

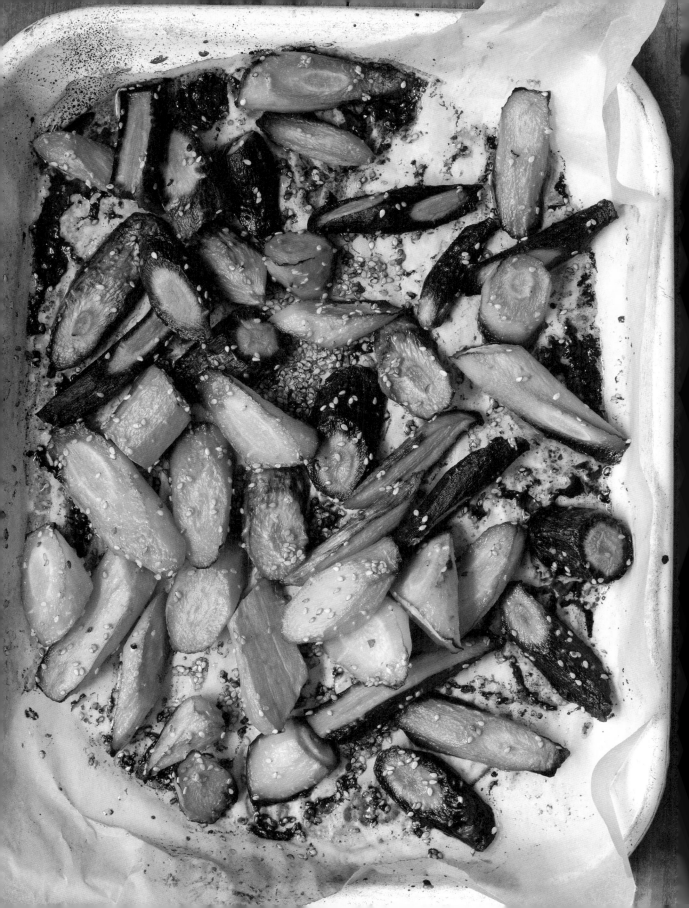

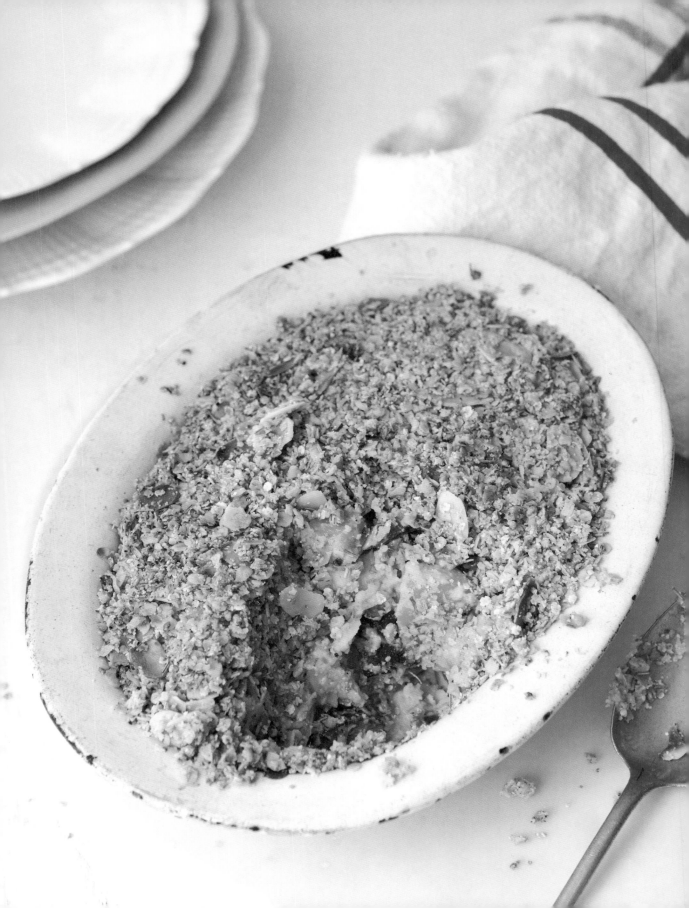

VEGETABLE CRUMBLE IN A CREAMY THYME SAUCE

If you fancy a change then this dish makes a great alternative to a Sunday roast. It's utterly delicious and satisfies every craving, even for a meat-eater!

serves 6

For the filling:

1½ tbsp goat's butter or vegan butter

2 cloves garlic, finely chopped

1 leek, finely chopped

½ cup carrot, cubed

¾ cup celeriac, cubed

½ cup roasted butternut squash, cubed

¼ cup zucchini, cubed

1 cup ceps or chanterelle mushrooms, chopped

1 tbsp chopped fresh flat-leaf parsley

For the white sauce:

3 tbsp goat's butter or vegan butter

⅓ cup rice flour

1¼ cups unsweetened rice or oat milk, warmed

1 sprig thyme

Himalayan pink salt and cracked black pepper, to season

For the crumble:

3½ tbsp goat's butter

generous 1 cup gluten-free oats

1 cup barley flakes

¼ cup slivered almonds

1 tsp dried rosemary

1 tsp Himalayan pink salt

Preheat the oven to 325°F.

If you don't have any roasted butternut squash, you'll need to roast some before starting the crumble. For this recipe, you'll need around 3½ oz of raw squash; peel, cut in half, and coat in 1 teaspoon of sunflower oil. Roast for 15 minutes. Remove from the oven and set aside.

Meanwhile, make the filling. Melt the butter in a pan over medium heat. Then, add the garlic and leek and sauté lightly for 1 minute.

Add the carrot, celeriac, and butternut squash and sauté for another 10 minutes on a low heat, adding 1 teaspoon of water every now and again to keep the temperature in the pan low. When the vegetables begin to soften, add the zucchini and mushrooms and sauté for another 4 minutes. Then set aside while you prepare the white sauce.

Next, make the sauce. In a separate pan, make a roux with the butter and the flour. Add the warmed milk slowly and keep stirring to combine until all the milk has been absorbed and the sauce reaches the desired consistency. Then pop in the thyme sprig and season to taste.

Move the vegetables into a baking dish, pour over the sauce, and combine well. Add the parsley.

Finally, make the crumble topping. Melt the butter in a large skillet. Add all the other ingredients and stir well to combine. Take off the heat and let it cool enough so you can squeeze the mixture between your fingers. Sprinkle the crumble on top of the creamy vegetables and bake in the preheated oven for 30 minutes.

I like to serve my crumble straight from the oven with blanched green beans and wilted spinach or a large fresh salad.

COCONUT RICE PUDDING

This is an old-fashioned favorite in need of a revamp and return to glory, and what better way than to make an Honestly Healthy version? And it's not like the one you used to have at school, we promise! This version is deliciously comforting. Just increase the quantities to serve up for a family lunch or tuck in after a midweek dinner à deux.

serves 2

⅓ cup short-grain brown rice

generous ¾ cup coconut milk

1 cup water

1 tsp dry unsweetened coconut

½ vanilla bean, split and scraped

a pinch of nutmeg

1 tbsp coconut palm sugar

1 tbsp dairy-free coconut cream

seeds and pulp of 1 passionfruit or date syrup
  and ground cinnamon, for topping

Preheat the oven to 325°F.

Put the uncooked rice into a high-speed blender and whiz for 15 seconds, until it begins to break up a little—do not over-blend, though, as the grains will become too fine.

Put the blitzed rice into a nonstick, lidded ovenproof pan followed by half the coconut milk and half the water, the dry unsweetened coconut, seeds from the vanilla bean, nutmeg, and palm sugar. Mix the ingredients together until well combined. Put the lid on and place in the oven. After 10 minutes stir and then replace the lid and return to the oven.

After 20 minutes add the other half of the water and coconut milk, stir well, and carry on cooking with the lid on, stirring every 10 minutes until it's been in the oven for 40 minutes. Remove from the oven and stir in the coconut cream.

Serve hot with a topping of passionfruit, or if you are feeling indulgent, a sprinkling of cinnamon and a drizzle of date syrup.

TASH'S TIPS

I find using a nonstick pan really helps the rice pudding to stay wet rather than burning the bottom of the pan. Be sure to use oven mitts or a dishtowel when you take the pan out of the oven as it will be really hot.

NUTRITIONAL NUGGET

Coconut cream is high in calcium for bone health, and zinc to boost immunity—a little goes a long way!

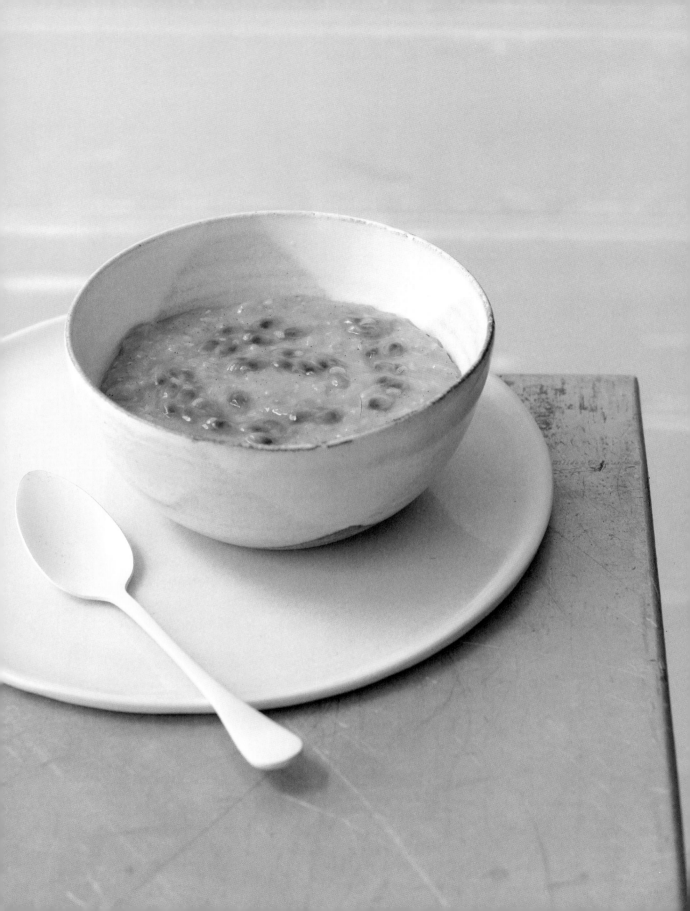

MOVIE NIGHT

CRUNCHY TOFFEE POPCORN

When you think of movies, popcorn somehow springs to mind. So why not make some for an at-home film night? Make sure you source organic, non-GM corn kernels; genetically modified food is a no-no in the Honestly Healthy world of eating. Now, sit back, enjoy, and watch the movie.

serves 4

1 tbsp sunflower oil

5 tbsp corn kernels

generous ⅓ cup coconut palm sugar

scant ½ cup agave syrup

1 tbsp vegan butter

a pinch of Himalayan pink salt

Preheat the oven to 212°F, and line a baking sheet with parchment paper.

Heat the sunflower oil in a large lidded pan, add the corn kernels, replace the lid, and leave the corn to pop over medium heat. Transfer the popcorn to a large mixing bowl.

Now make the caramel. Put a nonstick pan over medium heat and add the coconut palm sugar and agave syrup. Once the coconut palm sugar has dissolved into the agave, add the butter and salt to it to make it a little creamier. This entire process should take around 5 to 7 minutes.

Pour the caramel over the popcorn and mix well, ensuring that all the popcorn is coated.

Lay the caramel-coated popcorn on the prepared baking sheet and bake in the preheated oven for 30 minutes to dry out. Keep a close eye on it to make sure it does not burn.

Serve in a large bowl for everyone to share or make up some fun paper cones.

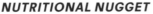

NUTRITIONAL NUGGET
Homemade popcorn is packed with cancer-preventing polyphenols— and fiber, too.

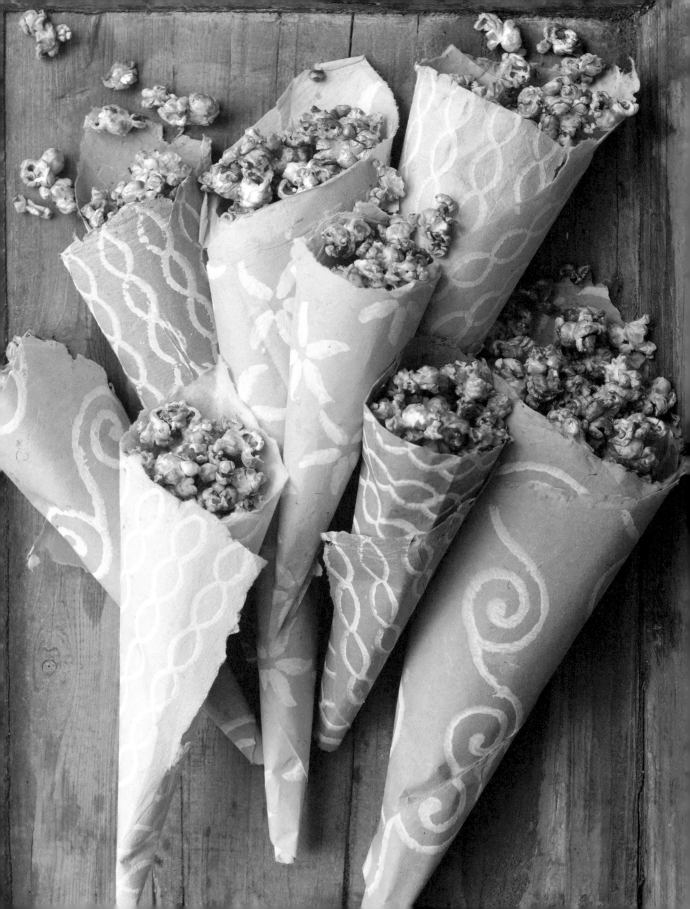

SESAME BURGERS

These veggie burgers could fool any beef-burger junky and are perfect to eat while watching a movie. Keep leftovers in the refrigerator in an airtight container and take to work for lunch the next day. They work especially well with a spicy salsa, so if you're inclined that way, rustle one up.

makes 6 burgers

2½ tbsp sunflower oil, plus extra for sautéing
½ small red onion, thinly sliced
a pinch of Himalayan pink salt
1 eggplant, cut into ½-in cubes
1 large vine tomato, thinly sliced
14 oz canned chickpeas, rinsed and drained
½ clove garlic, grated
1 small carrot, very thinly sliced or grated
3 tbsp cilantro, chopped
1¾ cups oats
¾ cup sesame seeds, for coating

For the yogurt dressing:
1 tsp cilantro, chopped
finely grated lemon zest of ¼ lemon
scant ½ cup goat's or sheep's yogurt
   (use a dairy-free version to keep this entire
   recipe vegan)

In a pan, heat 2 tablespoons of sunflower oil over medium heat. Add the onion and a pinch of salt and sauté for 2 minutes. Next, add the eggplant. After around 3 minutes, when the oil has been absorbed, add ½ tablespoon of oil and cook for another 5 minutes before adding the tomato. Next, add the tomato and cook for another 2 to 3 minutes.

Put the chickpeas, eggplant mixture, grated garlic, and carrots into a blender. Pulse until you have a rough mixture.

Transfer the mixture from the blender into a bowl and add the chopped cilantro and oats. Mix together well and then shape into patties in your hand; I make mine around 3¼ inches across and ½-inch thick. Roll each patty in sesame seeds and then sauté in sunflower oil for 1 to 2 minutes on each side, until golden brown.

Make the yogurt dressing by mixing together the ingredients and—hey presto—you have a fabulously fresh dipping sauce.

Serve the burgers with the yogurt sauce and a big vibrant salad.

TASH'S TIPS
If you soak eggplant in water for an hour before you want to use them, they will need much less oil during cooking.

NUTRITIONAL NUGGET
Chickpeas are packed with fiber to help reduce carbohydrate cravings and lower the incidence of potential diabetes. They are also a great source of manganese, essential for bone and ligament health.

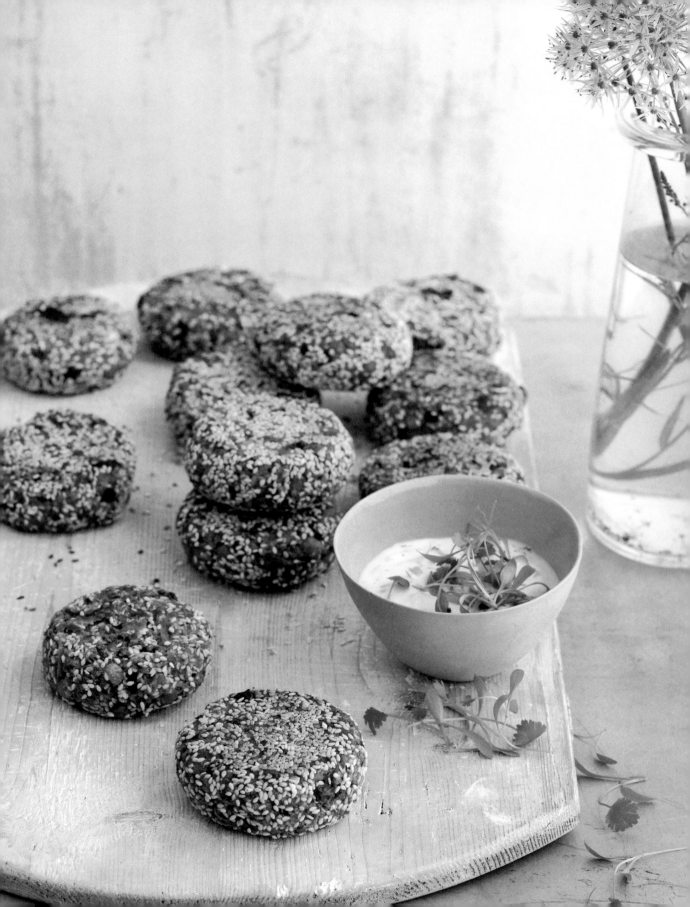

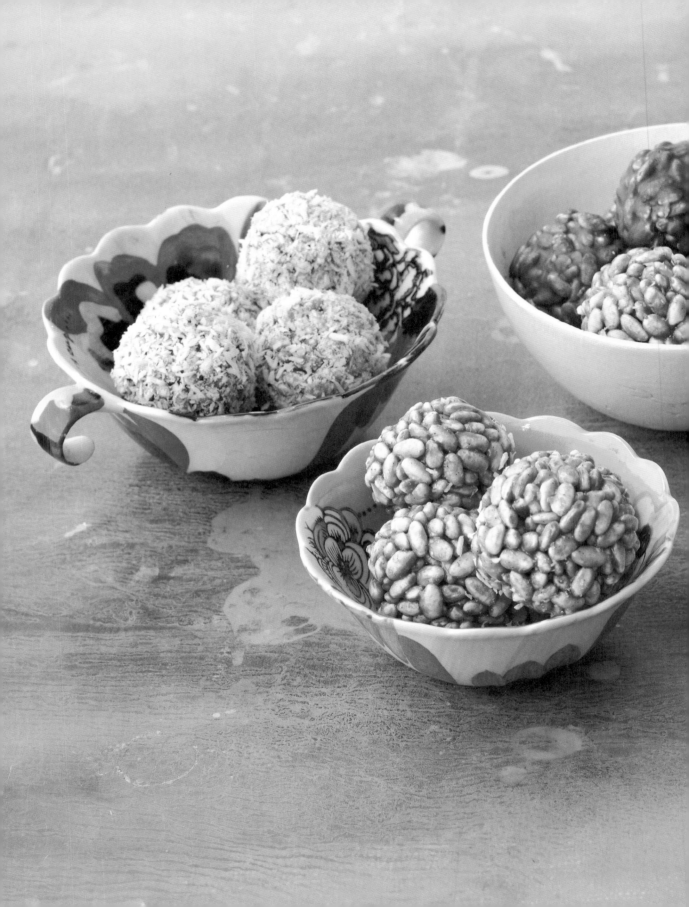

RICE POP BALLS

Kids—big and small—love these sweet little treats.
You can whip up these ridiculously tasty balls at a
moment's notice. And then just pop in the mouth.

makes 20 balls

⅓ cup sesame seed paste

3 tbsp date syrup

2 tsp vanilla extract

2 tbsp agave syrup

1 tbsp raw cacao powder

½ tsp cinnamon

finely grated zest of 1 orange

3½ cups unsweetened puffed rice

dry unsweetened coconut, crushed nuts, or
  grated raw cacao, to coat

Place all the ingredients apart from the puffed rice
in a large bowl and mix thoroughly with a spatula
until you have a smooth paste. Add the puffed rice
and stir until all the rice is well coated and sticky.

Put a heaping tablespoon of the mixture into the
palm of your hand and roll into a ball. Wash your
hands in between rolling each ball otherwise the
balls will fall apart.

Once all the balls are formed, you can roll them in
your choice of coating to jazz them up a little or just
leave them plain—they're delicious whichever way
you choose.

Mango Smash

I find the Indian Alphonso mango is the best for
this drink—it's packed with vitamin C and beta-
carotene and its juiciness and "perfumed" taste
is a crowd pleaser.

MAKES 4 SMALL OR 2 LARGE GLASSES

4 Alphonso mangoes, skin and stone
  removed

1 medium orange, juiced

2 limes, juiced

2 apples, juiced

1 small bunch of mint leaves

4 shots vodka or gin (optional)

Combine all the ingredients in a blender, adding
2 or 3 cubes of ice to dilute, as required. Serve
immediately.

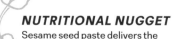

TASH'S TIPS

Washing your hands between rolling
really does help to keep the balls
together. The warmer your hands, the
less they will form into balls.

NUTRITIONAL NUGGET

Sesame seed paste delivers the
immune-boosting mineral selenium,
which also boosts metabolism.

MELT-IN-THE-MOUTH DONUTS

Close your eyes and sink your teeth into these baked donuts—yes, baked! These are not as light and fluffy as store-bought versions, but I think they're fabulous—perfect for a movie night. The frosting on page 179 makes a great alternative glaze, too.

makes 4 to 6 large donuts

For the donuts:
½ cup brown rice flour
¼ cup millet flour
2 tbsp potato flour
2 tbsp almond milk powder or soy milk powder
1 tbsp tapioca flour
½ tsp xanthan gum
1 tsp baking powder
¼ tsp Himalayan pink salt
½ cup coconut palm sugar
scant ¼ cup sunflower oil
2 large eggs
scant ¼ cup almond milk
1 tsp vanilla extract

For the glaze:
½ cup agave sugar
2 tbsp almond milk
½ tsp vanilla extract
½ tsp ground cinnamon

Preheat the oven to 325°F, and you'll also need a donut oven tin.

Sift all the dry ingredients (from brown rice flour to coconut palm sugar) together in a bowl.

In another bowl, whisk all the wet ingredients (from sunflower oil to vanilla extract) together until smooth. Then add the dry ingredients into the wet ingredients and mix. Mix thoroughly until all the ingredients are well combined. It is a really sticky batter and rather difficult to handle, so the easiest way to "tray" them up is to transfer the batter into a pastry bag.

Pipe the batter into the donut tin or carefully into loose rings (keeping the size of a shot glass hole in the middle). Bake for 12 to 15 minutes, or until golden.

Meanwhile, make the glaze. First sift the agave sugar into a bowl, then add the almond milk, vanilla extract, and cinnamon, stir until smooth, and set aside.

Remove the donuts from the oven and let cool on a wire rack. When completely cool, pour or brush on the glaze. These are best eaten on the same day—which I've never found to be a problem!

NUTRITIONAL NUGGET
Millet flour is one of the most nutrient-dense grains, rich in tryptophan and magnesium, both of which help boost mood.

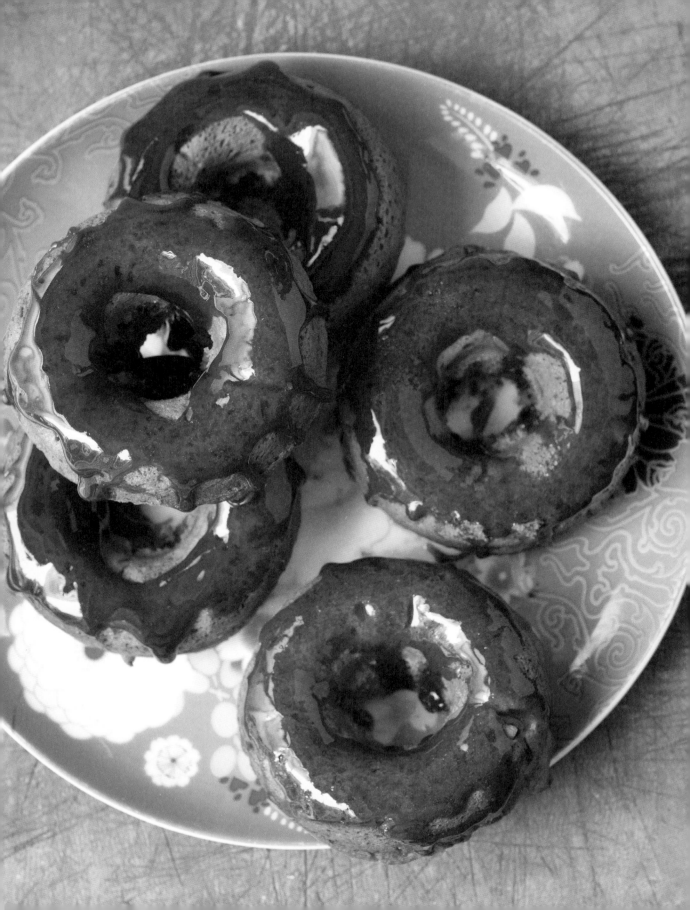

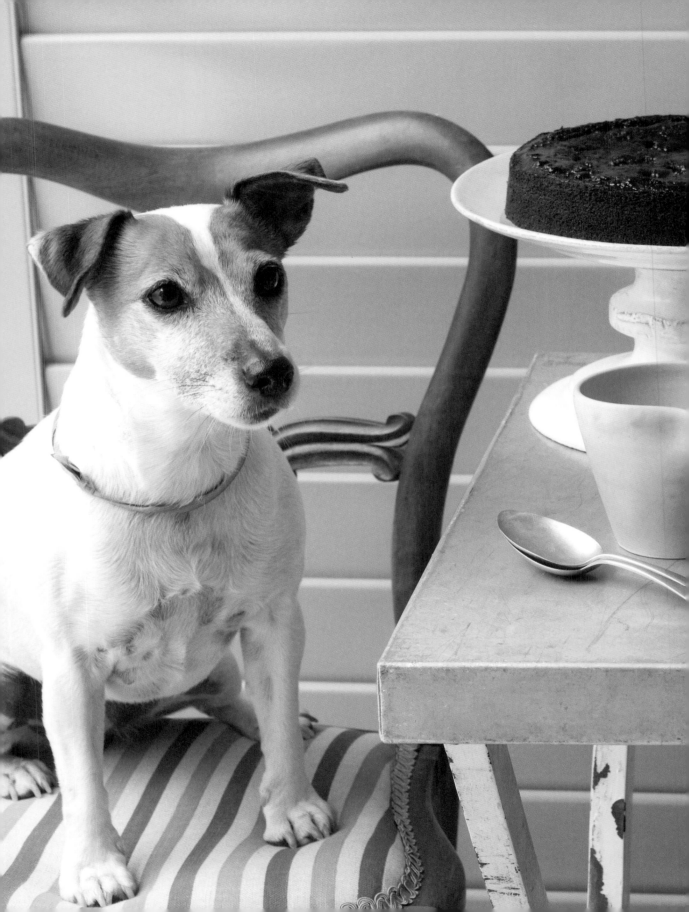

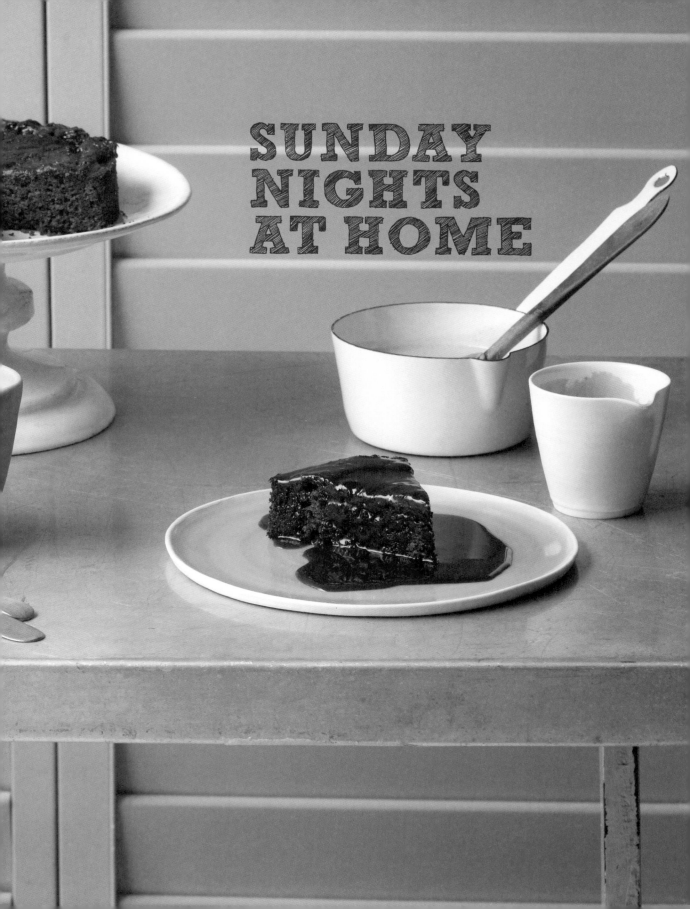

SUNDAY
NIGHTS
AT HOME

TANDOORI BITES

A healthy way to get the flavors of the Indian tandoori style of cooking to your table, I like to serve these as little pre-dinner bites. Change the yogurt in the sauce to dairy-free if you want it all to be vegan.

serves 3/makes 9 balls

For the tandoori sauce:
1 tsp turmeric
1 tsp cayenne pepper
1 tsp ground coriander
1 tsp ground ginger
1 tsp fennel seeds
1 tsp sweet paprika
1 tsp ground cumin
a pinch of Himalayan pink salt

For the bites:
1½ oz plain tofu
1 cup ground almonds
⅓ cup cilantro, chopped

For the dipping sauce:
½ cup goat's or sheep's yogurt
juice of ½ lime
½ tbsp rice wine vinegar
½ clove garlic

Preheat the oven to 325°F, and line a baking sheet with parchment paper.

For the tandoori sauce, simply blend all the spices and salt together and transfer to a shallow bowl and set aside.

In another bowl, use your hands to break up the tofu so that it looks "scrambled" and then add the ground almonds (keeping 2 tablespoons aside for the coating). Spoon in 2 tablespoons of the tandoori sauce along with the chopped cilantro and mix until well combined.

Roll the mixture into ping-pong-sized balls, then roll the balls into the remaining tandoori sauce (keep any leftover sauce for dipping later) and then again into the almonds. Arrange the balls on the prepared tray and bake in a preheated oven for 15 minutes, or until just going golden and crispy on the outside.

To make the dipping sauce, simply combine all the ingredients in a small bowl.

Serve the tandoori balls hot or cold with the zingy dipping sauce and any leftover tandoori sauce on the side.

TASH'S TIPS
If you find your mixture is a bit too wet, then add more ground almonds to the mixture to help bind it together.

NUTRITIONAL NUGGET
Turmeric, cayenne, coriander, and fennel seeds provide immune-stimulating, metabolism-enhancing, and digestive-supporting nutrients—all power to the Asian spices!

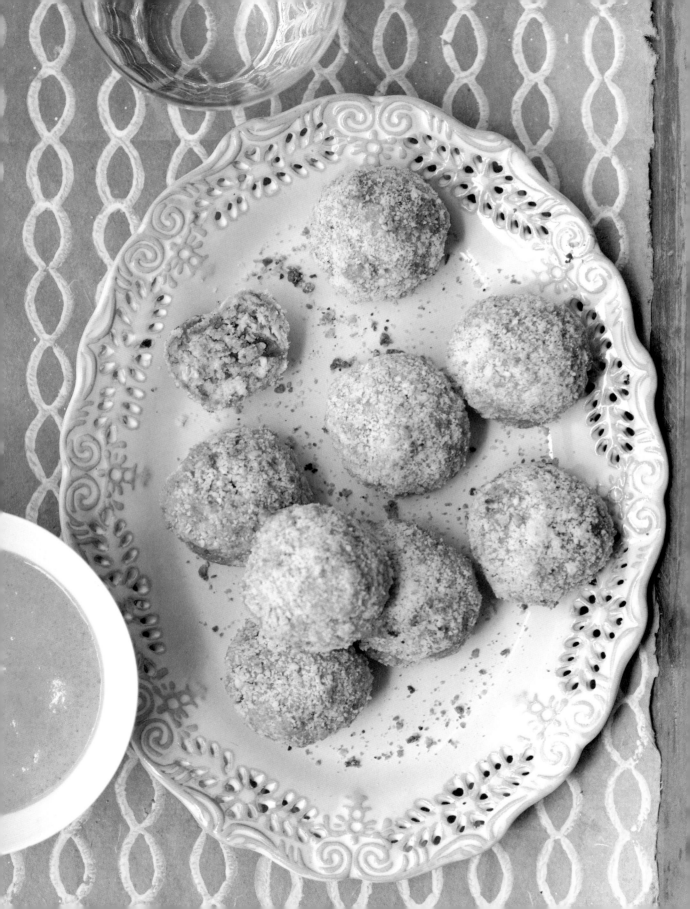

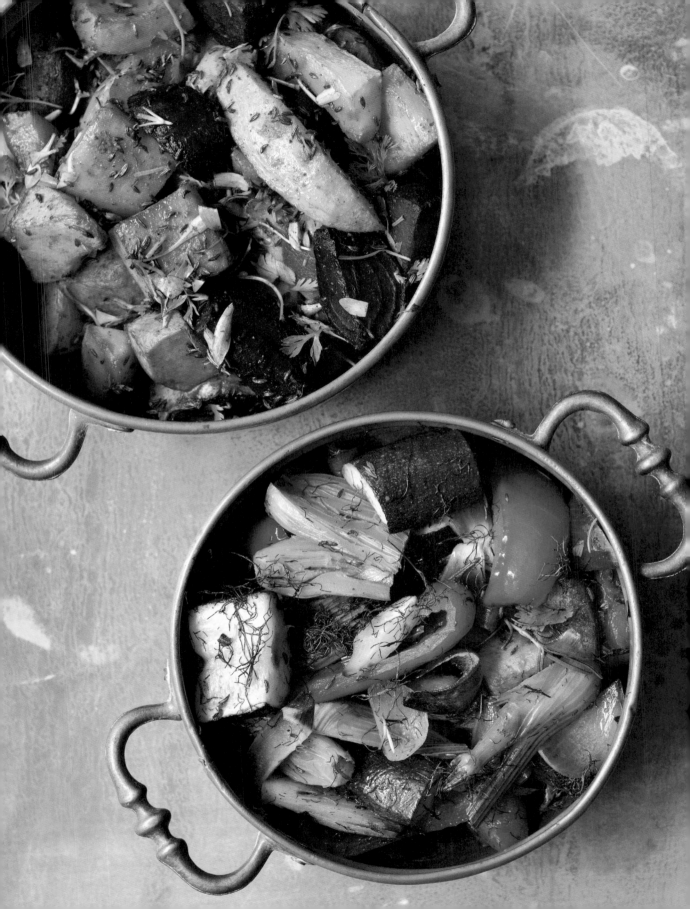

MASALA ROASTED ROOT VEGETABLES

*I love Indian food, but sometimes don't fancy a full-
on curry, so this is a way to have a taste of Indian
cuisine without having a heavy meal. It's a delicious
partner to a salad or a side dish to a dhal.*

serves 4 as a side dish

For sheet 1:

½ small butternut squash (around 6½ oz),
   peeled and cut into ¾ x 1¼-in chunks

2 medium beets (around 6½ oz), peeled and
   cut into ½ x ¾-in chunks

1 medium sweet potato (around 6½ oz), peeled
   and cut into ¾ x 1¼-in chunks

½ tsp garam masala

¼ tsp smoked paprika

2 tsp caraway seeds

¼ tsp Himalayan pink salt

1 tbsp sunflower oil

For sheet 2:

1 zucchini (around 6½ oz), trimmed and cut
   into ¾ x 1¼-in chunks

1 large red bell pepper (around 5½ oz), cut into
   ¾-in cubes

1 red onion

¼ tsp nutmeg

3 sprigs of thyme

¼ tsp Himalayan pink salt

1 tbsp sunflower oil

To serve:

3 tbsp cilantro (or other herbs), chopped
finely grated zest of ½ lemon

Preheat the oven to 350°F. You'll need two large
baking sheets.

Do one sheet at a time. Start with sheet 1. When the
vegetables are prepped, place them in a mixing
bowl with the spices, salt, and oil. Mix thoroughly
with your hands, transfer to the baking sheet, and
pop in the preheated oven for 20 minutes.

For sheet 2, again prep the vegetables and mix
thoroughly in a bowl with the spice, herbs, salt, and
oil. Roast for 15 minutes alongside the other sheet
of vegetables.

When both sheets of vegetables are cooked, mix
them together in a large serving dish (or serve
each separately if you wish). Sprinkle some
chopped fresh herbs—cilantro works well—over
the top, grate some lemon zest over it, and mix
through.

You can vary the vegetables depending on what
you have lying around—they always taste delicious
when combined with the spices.

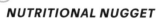

NUTRITIONAL NUGGET
Beet is a great source of iron
and vitamin C, as well as
magnesium—great for relaxing
and calming the mind.

WILD MUSHROOM QUINOA "RISOTTO"

This was an amazing accident on a Sunday when I had no brown rice to make a risotto, so I reached for the quinoa and this delicious concoction ended up on my plate. Feel free to use different veggies if you want to experiment or don't have these on hand.

serves 3 to 4

1 tbsp sunflower oil

3 cloves garlic, sliced

2½ cups boiling water, plus extra scant ¼ cup

1 tbsp bouillon powder

scant 1½ cups quinoa

7 oz wild mushrooms (some left whole, some sliced, and some cubed)

3 tbsp vegan butter

scant ¼ cup hard goat's cheese, grated

3 tbsp flat-leaf parsley, chopped

In a pan, heat the sunflower oil and 1 clove of garlic, finely chopped, over medium heat for around 1 minute, until soft.

Make the stock with 2½ cups boiling water and the bouillon powder and add to the pan along with the quinoa. After 5 minutes, add half the mushrooms and keep over medium heat, stirring frequently.

In a separate pan, melt 1 tablespoon of the vegan butter and add the remaining garlic cloves. Sauté the garlic until soft, add the remaining mushrooms, and continue to sauté for 3 to 4 minutes until soft and brown. Remove from the heat.

After 10 minutes of cooking, the quinoa should have absorbed all of the water—keep stirring and then add another scant ¼ cup of boiling water. Continue to stir as you would if making a normal risotto. After 20 minutes, add the grated goat's cheese and allow to melt, then take off the heat and put the lid on. Let it sit for 5 minutes.

In a small pan, melt the remaining vegan butter, then toss in the parsley and mix through.

To serve, add the remaining mushrooms to the "risotto" and, finally, pour over the parsley butter.

TASH'S TIPS
Try with asparagus and lemon instead of the mushrooms for an alternative flavor combination.

NUTRITIONAL NUGGET
Quinoa is actually a seed, rather than a grain, packed with protein and omega-3 for energy, while mushrooms boost immunity.

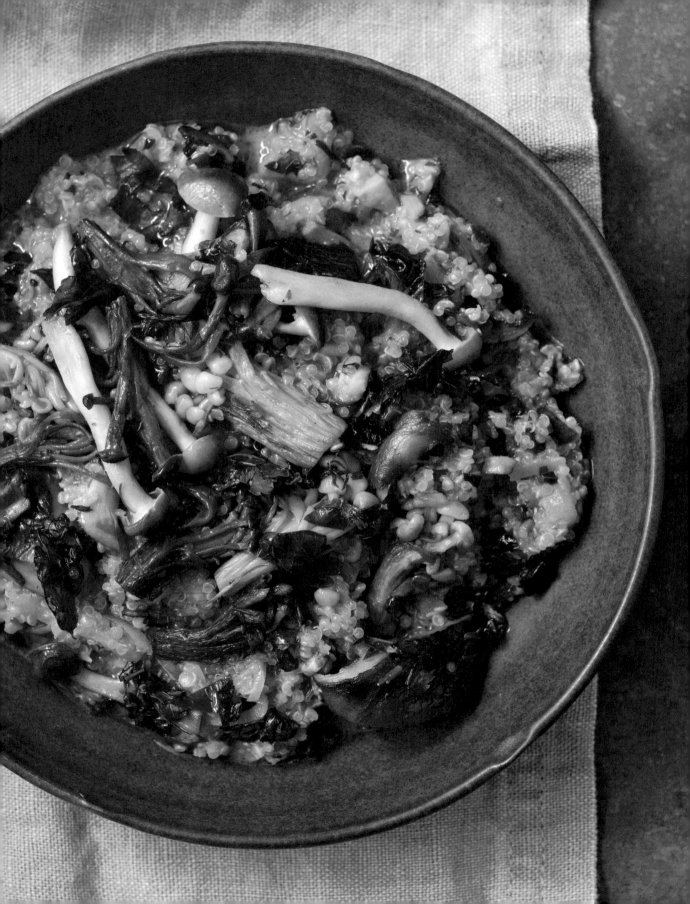

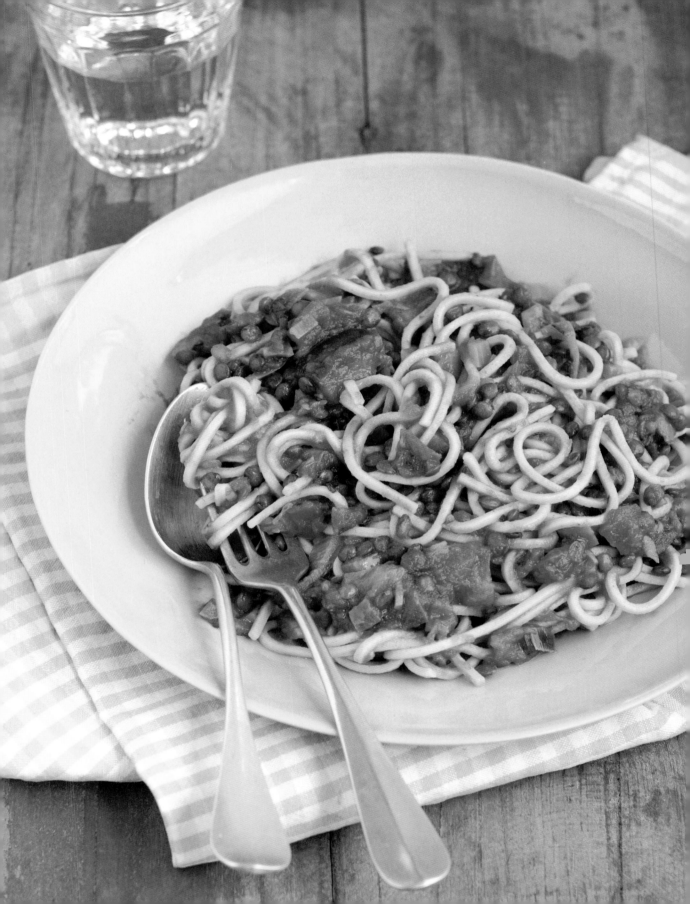

SIENNA'S SPAGHETTI BOLOGNAISE

*Growing up, my stepsister Sienna and I often had
"spag bol" after school and it was always the first
thing we used to order when we went on vacation.
Even today it's one of our favorites, and now I've
created this vegetarian version so we can continue
to enjoy it together.*

serves 6

3¾ cups water

1½ tbsp bouillon powder

2 tbsp sunflower oil, plus extra for drizzling

1 large white onion, chopped

1 red onion, finely chopped

2 cloves garlic, finely chopped

scant ½ cup water

8 vine tomatoes, chopped

2 bay leaves

1 tbsp cumin

½ eggplant, chopped into ¾-in cubes

1 cup Puy lentils

1 tsp balsamic vinegar

1 tsp tamari

a pinch of Himalayan pink salt

Preheat the oven to 350°F.

First, make the stock by boiling the measured
water and the bouillon powder in a pan. Heat until
the powder has dissolved, then set aside.

In a large pan, heat the sunflower oil with the
onions and garlic and sauté over medium heat for
2 to 3 minutes. Add scant ¼ cup of water and leave
to simmer until all the water is absorbed into the
onion—when this is done add the remaining water.

Next, add the vine tomatoes and bay leaves and let
the mixture sweat for 2 minutes. Add generous
1 cup of stock and the cumin and leave to simmer
over medium heat for 10 minutes. Add the eggplant
along with another 1¼ cups of stock. After
5 minutes, add the Puy lentils along with 1¼ cups
of stock and the balsamic vinegar.

Leave to cook for another 20 minutes and then add
the tamari. Taste and add salt if needed.

Remove the bay leaves and serve the lentil sauce
over gluten-free spaghetti.

TASH'S TIPS
If you like your sauce on the sloppy
side, then add ½ cup of fresh tomato
juice just before taking it off the stove.

NUTRITIONAL NUGGET
Puy lentils provide a good source of
iron, as well as fiber to regulate
elimination and prevent a host of
digestive complaints.

STICKY TOFFEE PUDDING AND CUSTARD

If you're longing for something decadent and rich, then give this recipe a try. It's one of my favorite desserts and is ridiculously easy to make. Enjoy with your family and friends, but remember— everything in moderation!

makes 8 to 10 slices

For the cake:
¼ cup raw cashew nuts (optional)
scant ½ cup vegan butter
⅓ cup coconut palm sugar
¼ cup rice syrup
2 eggs, beaten
scant ¼ cup warm water
generous ¾ cup rice flour
scant ½ cup cornstarch
1 tsp baking powder
1 tsp baking soda
7 oz dates, pitted
½ cup water
1 tbsp raw cacao powder

For the custard:
generous 2 cups soy milk
2 tsp vanilla extract
2 tbsp agave syrup
2 eggs
a pinch of nutmeg
2 tbsp cornstarch or kuzu
1 tbsp cold water

For the toffee sauce:
generous ⅓ cup vegan butter
scant ½ cup coconut palm sugar
scant ½ cup rice syrup

Preheat the oven to 350°F and grease and line an 8-inch round cake pan with parchment paper. In a bowl, cover the cashews with water and soak for 30 minutes, then drain.

Melt the butter, sugar, and rice syrup over a low heat in a pan. Let cool, until you can stick your finger in without burning, and add the eggs (if it's too hot, the eggs will scramble) and scant ¼ cup of warm water and mix until smooth.

Sift the flours together with the baking powder and baking soda into a bowl.

Put the dates along with ½ cup of water and the cashews in a blender and blend until very smooth. Add the cacao and pulse in. Add the contents of the blender into the buttery egg and mix until well combined. Fold in the dry ingredients. Transfer the batter into the prepared cake pan and bake in a preheated oven for 30 minutes, or until a knife inserted into the center comes out clean.

While the cake is baking, make the custard. Heat the milk in a pan with the vanilla extract and agave syrup over medium heat. Bring to almost boiling, then remove from the heat. Beat the eggs, nutmeg, and cornstarch in a stainless-steel mixing bowl until well combined. Pour the hot milk over the eggy mix and whisk in well. Next, pour the egg mixture back into the pan and cook over gentle heat for 10 minutes, stirring with a wooden spoon, until it thickens and coats the back of the spoon. Mix the kuzu with 1 tablespoon of cold water and combine with the custard. Continue to stir until thickened. Remove from the heat quickly and pour back into the mixing bowl. Whisk well to cool a little and smooth it out. If you see any lumps then strain through a strainer. It's now ready to use. (If you make the custard ahead of time, cover the surface with plastic wrap to avoid a skin forming.)

Remove the cake from the oven, let cool in the pan for 10 to 15 minutes, and transfer to a wire rack.

To make the toffee sauce, simply heat all the ingredients in a pan over medium heat. Serve the pudding with a drizzle of sauce and the custard.

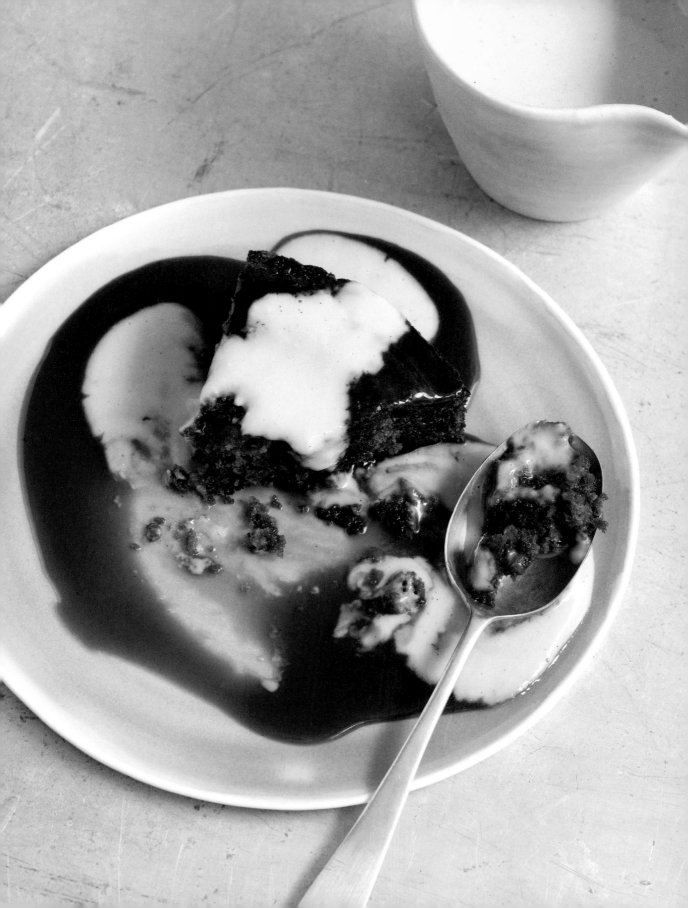

HELL OF A HULLABALOO

Who doesn't love a party or a celebratory gathering? I certainly do. Whether you're throwing a birthday party for children or adults, a get-together for one of the many events that mark our calendars (think Easter, Halloween, Thanksgiving, or Christmas), dip into this section for inspirational recipes on how to celebrate in style, the Honestly Healthy way.

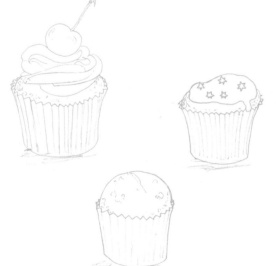

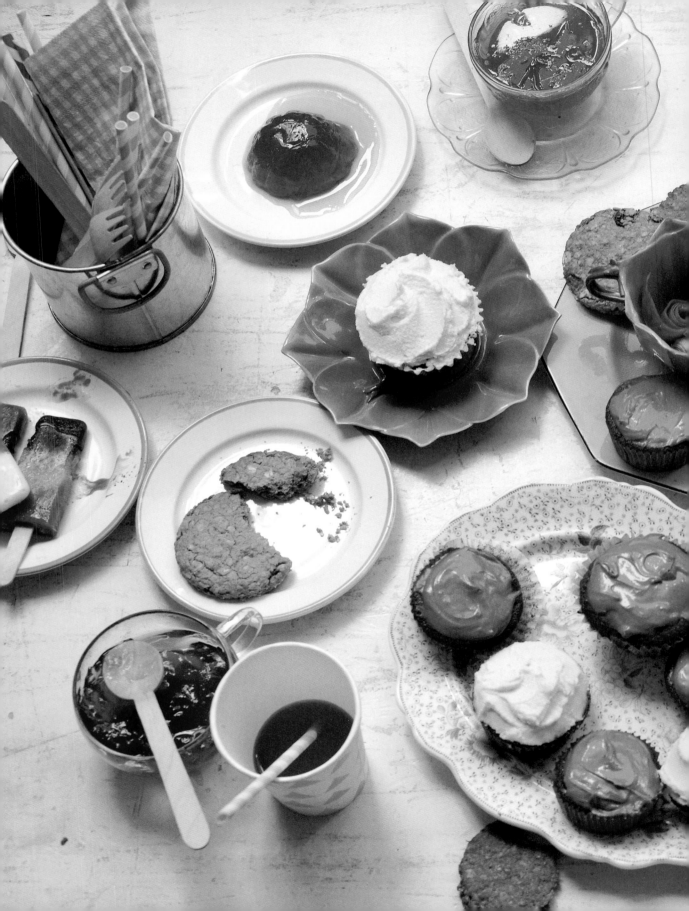

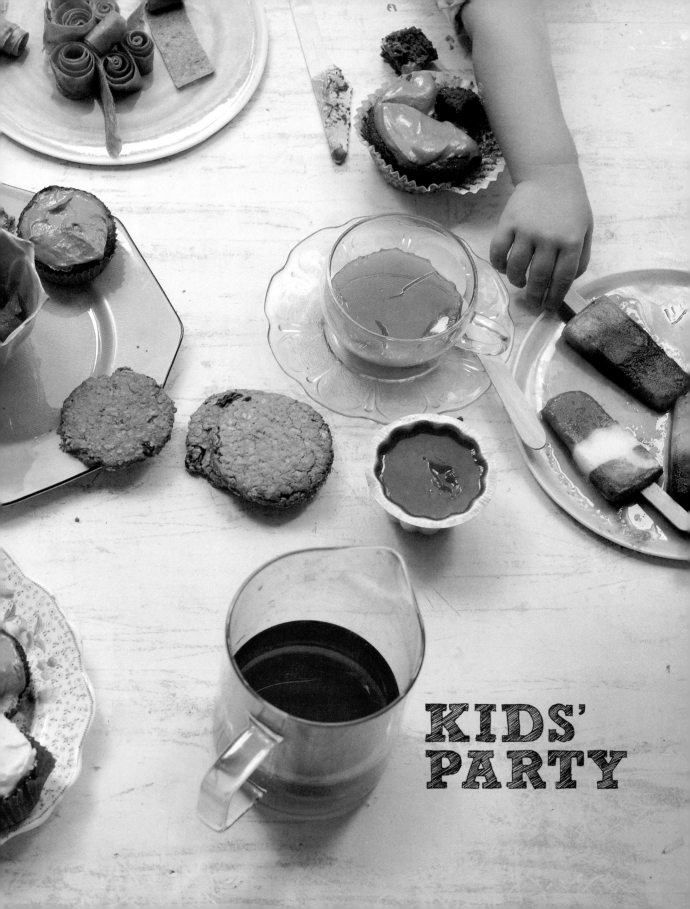

KIDS' PARTY

FRUITY ICE POPS

You can use whatever flavor combinations you like in these summery refreshers. Simply make fruit purées and freeze in molds. Enjoy mixing and matching flavor combinations.

♥ ♥

makes 6 to 8 ice pops

♥

4 ripe apricots, pitted
¼ cup alkaline or filtered water

♥

3 kiwi fruits, skins removed
3 tbsp mint, chopped
¼ cup alkaline or filtered water

1 cup blueberries
scant ½ cup goat's yogurt

♥

2¾ cups strawberries
¼ cup alkaline or filtered water

♥

1 banana
1 tbsp raw cashew nuts
scant ½ cup alkaline or
   filtered water

♥

14 oz pineapple, skin removed
⅓ cup alkaline or filtered water

Purée the ingredients for each flavor in a high-speed blender. Make each flavor separately, so that you have a palette of tastes to play with. And do rinse the blender in between.

Pour the purées into the ice pop holders as pure flavors, or layer them to create multi-striped tasty wonders. Freeze for 3 to 4 hours and then enjoy!

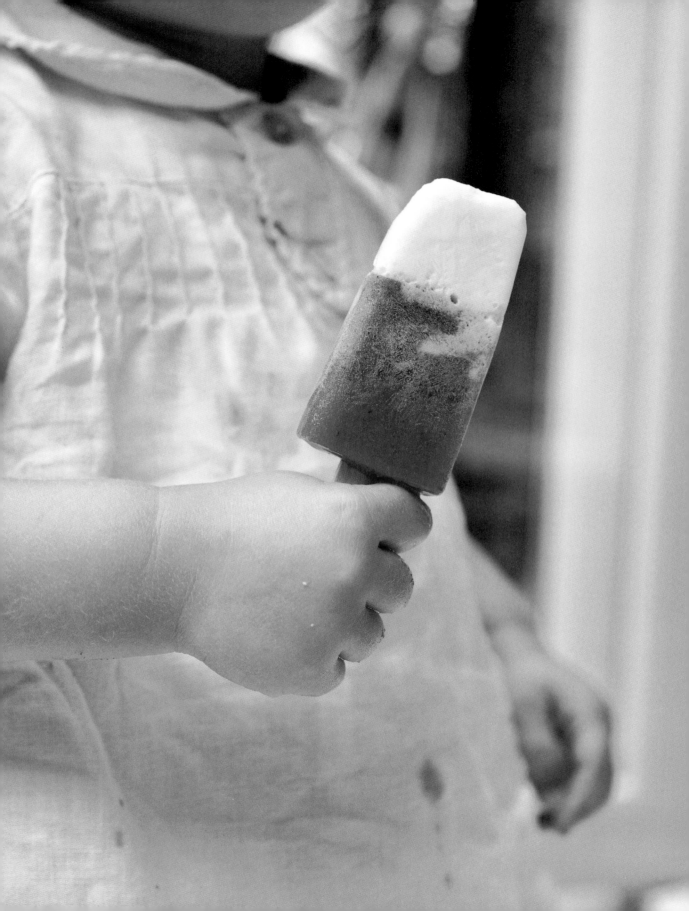

WIBBLY WOBBLY GELATIN

Everyone loves gelatin (even if it's when we are older and in a shot glass!), and these fruity numbers are a real crowd pleaser. You could add edible flowers for a delicate and beautiful dish. What's so great about making your own fresh gelatins is that you can change the flavor and the color by using different juices—and making the most of seasonal fruits. I press my own juices, but you can buy freshly pressed juices or unsweetened pure juices; I've found that teas can work well, too.

makes 4 to 6 small cups

generous 2 cups juice or liquid

4 tsp agar agar flakes

Pour the juice into a pan along with the agar agar. Bring it to a rolling boil and keep stirring until the agar agar has completely dissolved, which should take around 5 minutes. A white froth will develop on the surface of the hot liquid, but don't worry about that, just make sure you can't see any granules of agar agar.

Strain the contents of the pan through a strainer twice before transferring to your gelatin mold or bowl of choice. Some molds prove tricky in terms of getting agar agar gelatin out. You can line any molds with plastic wrap or set in pretty glasses for a dinner party.

Set in the refrigerator for 2 to 3 hours or, even better, overnight. Serve chilled.

TASH'S TIPS

Our favorite gelatin flavors are raspberry and apple, strawberry and lime, orange, apple and green tea, white grape and passionfruit, and cranberry and apple.

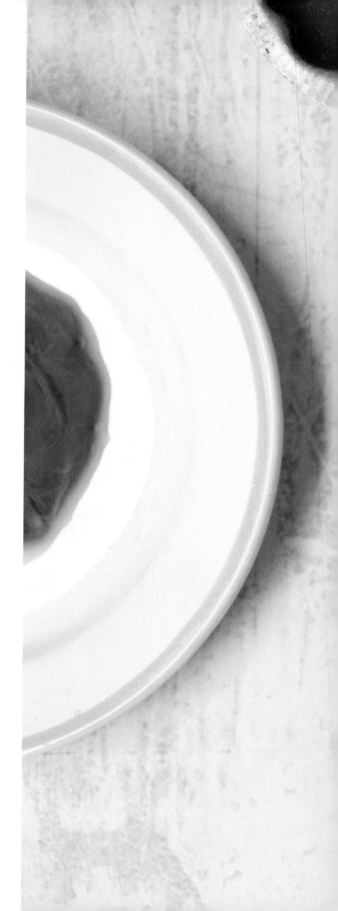

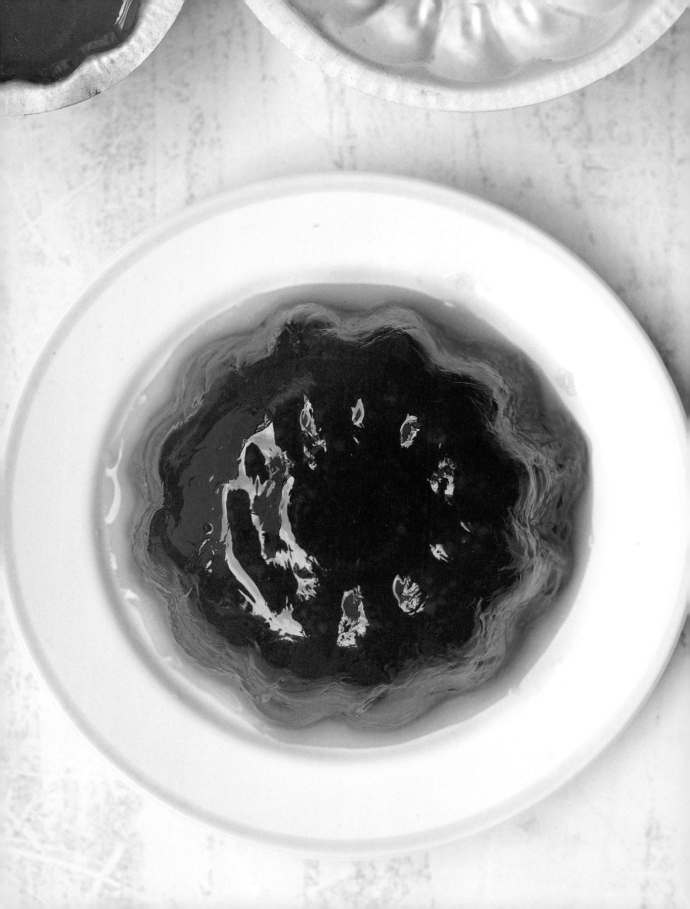

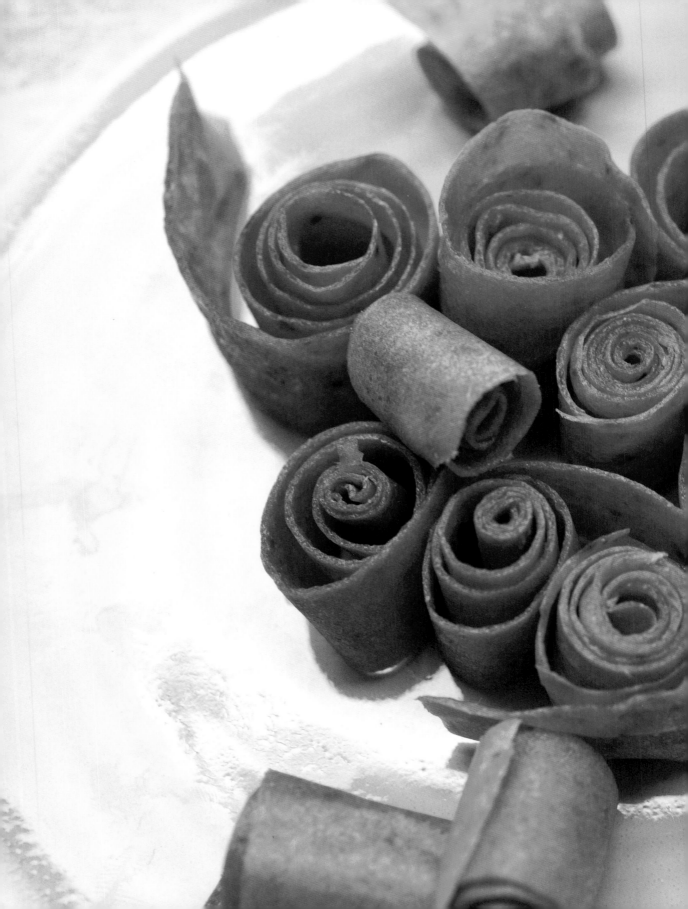

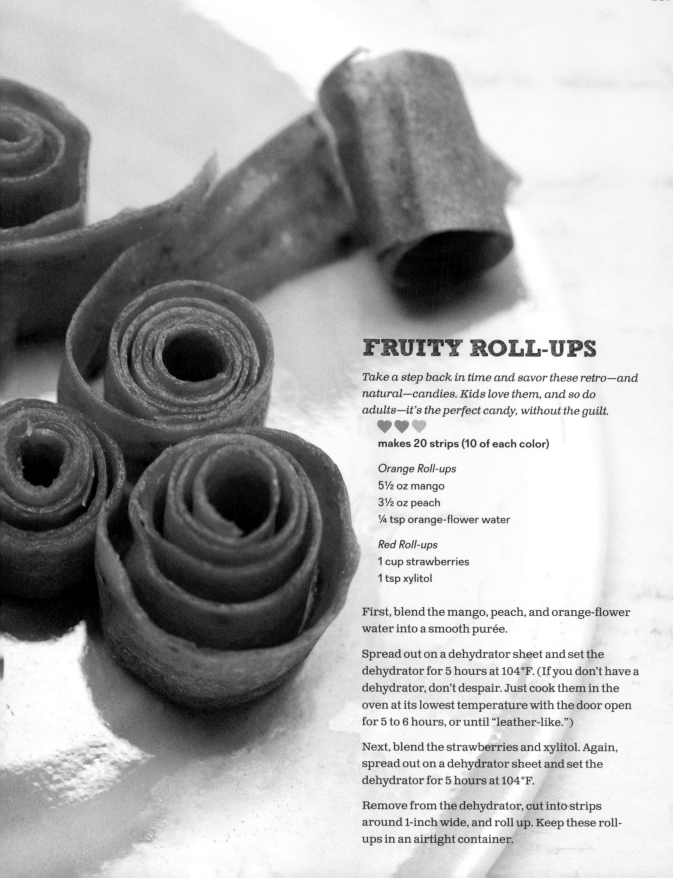

FRUITY ROLL-UPS

Take a step back in time and savor these retro—and natural—candies. Kids love them, and so do adults—it's the perfect candy, without the guilt.

♥ ♥ ♥

makes 20 strips (10 of each color)

Orange Roll-ups
5½ oz mango
3½ oz peach
¼ tsp orange-flower water

Red Roll-ups
1 cup strawberries
1 tsp xylitol

First, blend the mango, peach, and orange-flower water into a smooth purée.

Spread out on a dehydrator sheet and set the dehydrator for 5 hours at 104°F. (If you don't have a dehydrator, don't despair. Just cook them in the oven at its lowest temperature with the door open for 5 to 6 hours, or until "leather-like.")

Next, blend the strawberries and xylitol. Again, spread out on a dehydrator sheet and set the dehydrator for 5 hours at 104°F.

Remove from the dehydrator, cut into strips around 1-inch wide, and roll up. Keep these roll-ups in an airtight container.

RAISIN OAT COOKIES

Not just for kids, these are perfect for dunking into a cup of tea. But be warned—they are ridiculously tasty and addictive!

makes 12 to 16

generous 3 cups rice flour

2 tsp baking soda

2 tsp ground cinnamon

1 tsp ground ginger

1 tsp ground nutmeg

11 cups oats

1 cup vegan butter

2½ cups coconut palm sugar

4 eggs, beaten

2 tsp vanilla extract

1¾ cups raisins

Preheat the oven to 350°F and line a baking sheet with parchment paper.

In a bowl, mix the flour, baking soda, spices, and oats and combine well.

In a separate large bowl, beat together the butter, sugar, eggs, and vanilla extract. (Don't worry if your mixture looks like it's split, once the dried ingredients are mixed in it all comes together.)

Mix the dry ingredients into the wet mixture and add the raisins. Add extra raisins or oats if the mixture seems a little too wet, although the mixture is supposed to be quite sticky. Place tablespoons of the mixture on the baking sheet 1 inch apart and flatten slightly.

Bake for 10 to 15 minutes, then remove from the oven, transfer to a wire rack, and leave to cool.

TASH'S TIPS
If you want to make them a little more indulgent, add some sugar-free vegan chocolate chips or some pumpkin and sunflower seeds.

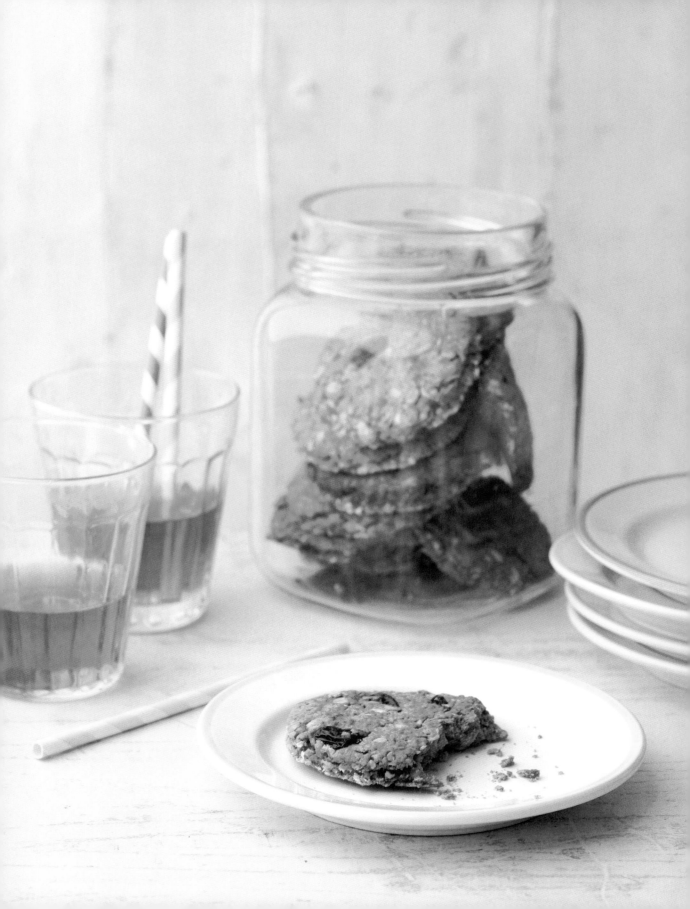

CUPCAKES

Everyone loves a cupcake and these light and fluffy mouthfuls could easily be baked as a whole cake. You'll need to make the frosting the day before, but you can throw these cupcakes together in no time. And if you like, you could always use the banoffee pie cream (see page 171), the gingerbread frosting (see page 179), or the chocolate frosting (see page 161)—which all work perfectly with these little cakes.

makes 18

1¼ cups rice milk

3 tbsp apple cider vinegar

½ cup oat flour (or blend your own oats)

scant 1 cup brown rice flour

½ cup tapioca flour

1 tsp xanthan gum

1 tsp baking soda

1 tsp baking powder

3 tbsp raw cacao powder

⅛ tsp Himalayan pink salt

1 cup vegan butter

¼ cup agave syrup

generous 1 cup coconut palm sugar

2 eggs

3 tbsp soy yogurt

1 tsp vanilla extract

⅓ cup beet juice

Preheat the oven to 350°F, and pop 18 paper liners into two 12-hole muffin pans.

First, make your homemade rice buttermilk. Mix the rice milk with the apple cider vinegar. Do not stir it; leave it to "ferment" for 15 minutes. This creates a substitute for buttermilk.

Sift the flours, xanthan gum, baking soda, baking powder, cacao powder, and salt together in a large mixing bowl.

Beat together the butter, agave, and coconut palm sugar until light and fluffy, then add the eggs, soy yogurt, vanilla extract, and the rice buttermilk you made at the start. Beat until well combined.

The batter might look like it has split, but don't worry. Slowly incorporate the dry mixture into the wet mixture (with a wooden spoon or on a low speed with an electric mixer) and watch as the batter comes together. Finally, add the beet juice.

The batter should have a heavy mousse-like texture. Spoon 2 heaping tablespoons of batter into each cupcake liner and bake in a preheated oven for 20 to 25 minutes.

Remove from the oven and allow them to cool completely before frosting them.

Super-tasty frosting for cupcakes

makes enough for 18 cupcakes

1½ cups coconut oil

1½ cups rice milk

½ cup dairy-free milk powder (almond or soy)

scant ¼ cup agave syrup

¼ cup coconut flour

1 tbsp vanilla extract

1 tbsp lemon juice

Melt the coconut oil in a heatproof bowl over a pan of simmering water (or a bain marie). Once melted, set aside.

Put the rice milk, milk powder, agave, coconut flour, and vanilla extract into a blender and whiz until well mixed and smooth. Add any colorings at this point. To make different colored frostings: add beet juice for pink, spirulina or chlorophyll for green, and turmeric for yellow. Just add a little at a time while blending to get the desired color.

Next, slowly add the slightly cooled coconut oil and the lemon juice and mix well. Transfer the contents into a bowl and refrigerate overnight.

While your cupcakes are cooling, take the bowl out of the refrigerator and allow it to soften up a bit, so it's malleable and easier to ice the cupcakes with.

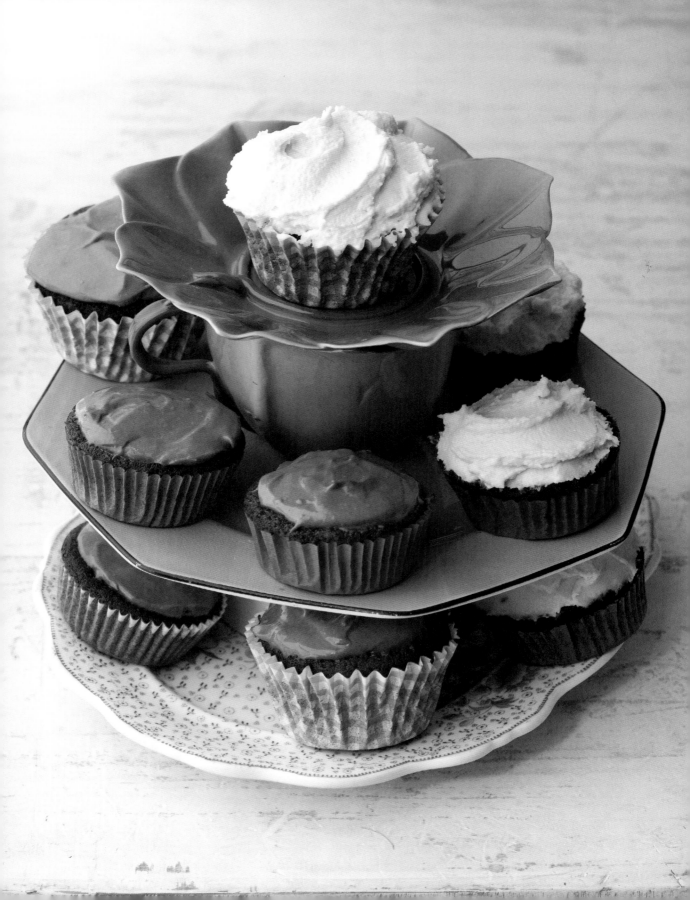

HALLOWEEN

BEET SOUP

Serve up this perfect blood red appetizer for your guests at Halloween—the color is so utterly gorgeous and the taste is devilishly good.

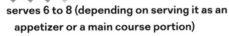

serves 6 to 8 (depending on serving it as an appetizer or a main course portion)

1 tbsp bouillon powder

2½ cups boiling water

2¼ lb beet

2 white onions

1 clove garlic

1 tbsp sunflower oil

1 tsp dried mixed herbs

1 tsp fennel seeds

3½ cups coconut milk

1 tsp umeboshi plum purée

1 tbsp apple cider vinegar

¾ oz tarragon leaves

Add the bouillon powder to the boiling water to make a vegetable stock and give it a good stir, until all the powder has dissolved. Set aside.

Peel the beet and chop into ¾-inch cubes, and finely chop the onion and garlic.

Heat the sunflower oil in a pan on a low heat. Add the onions and garlic and sauté together, then add the mixed herbs and the fennel seeds.

Once the onions have sweated off, add the beet cubes and the vegetable stock. Bring to a boil and then simmer for 20 minutes before adding the coconut milk and cooking for another 15 minutes.

Take the pan off the heat and let cool for 10 minutes before transferring the contents to a blender. Blend the soup into a smooth purée.

Add the umeboshi plum purée, vinegar, and half of the tarragon, and blend again.

Serve piping hot and garnish with the rest of the tarragon, if you like.

TASH'S TIPS

For a super-quick version of this soup, use boiled prepackaged beets and boil only for 5–10 minutes, following the first steps of the recipe.

NUTRITIONAL NUGGET

Apple cider vinegar helps to stimulate your stomach acid, so that it performs at its best in breaking down food, thereby allowing better absorption of nutrients further down the gut.

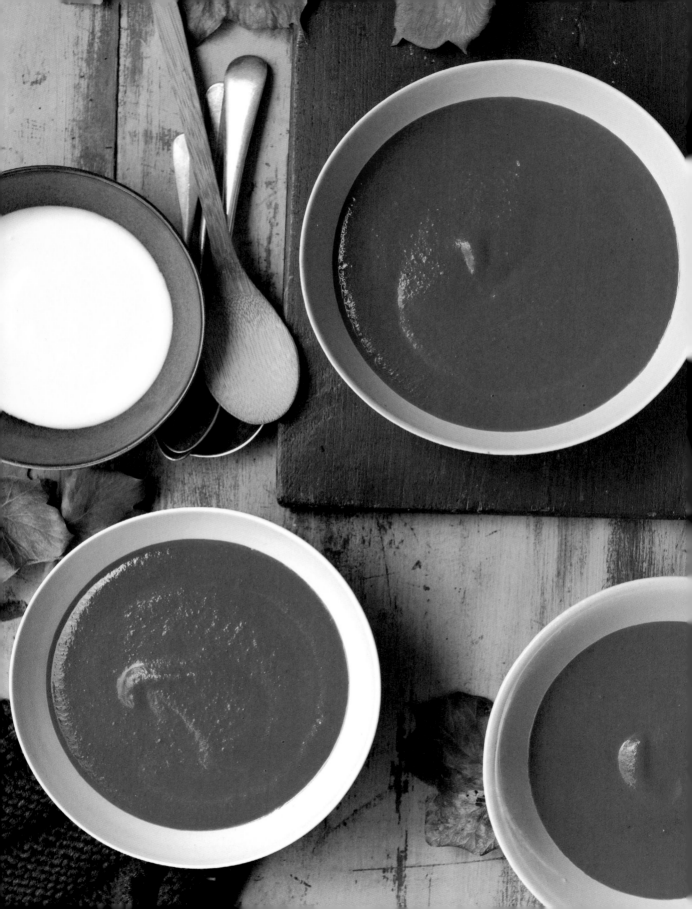

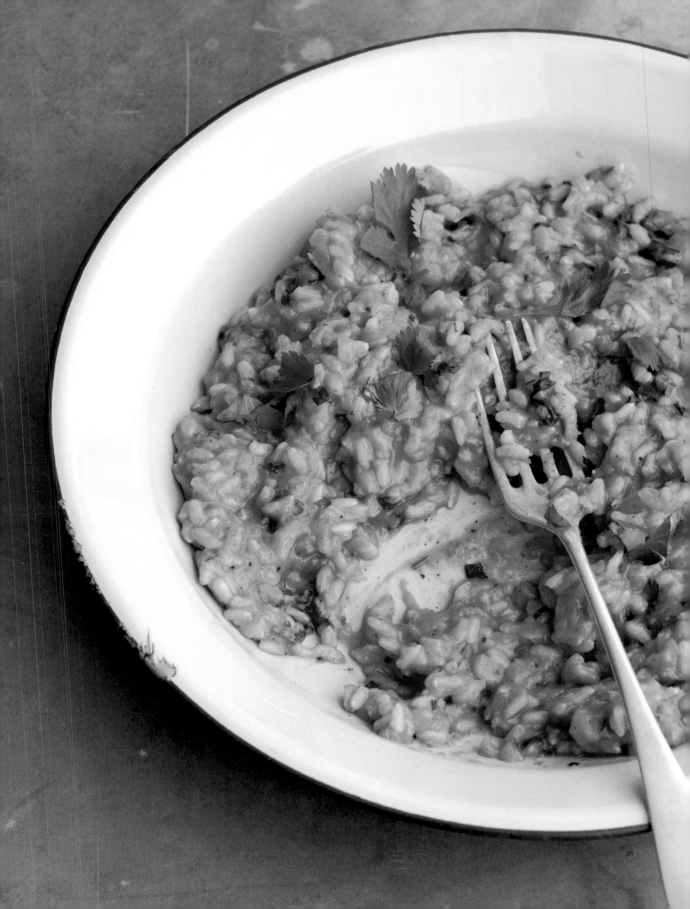

PUMPKIN AND ORANGE RISOTTO

It's pumpkins galore around Halloween, and I love them. Their sweetness adds a wonderful indulgence to any meal and this risotto is no exception. The super-smooth pumpkin purée is a partnership made in heaven with the brown risotto rice (don't worry if you don't have risotto rice, you can always use short grain brown rice).

serves 4

For the pumpkin purée:
10½ oz pumpkin, peeled and chopped into chunks
1 sprig of rosemary
1 tbsp sunflower oil

For the risotto:
8 cups water
1 heaping tsp bouillon powder
1 star anise
4 tsp sunflower oil
1 onion, finely chopped
1 clove garlic, finely chopped
1 tsp za'atar
¾ cup brown risotto rice
⅓ cup fresh orange juice
1½ cups pumpkin purée
⅓ cup flat-leaf parsley or cilantro, chopped, to garnish
a squeeze of lemon, to serve

For the caramelized onions:
4 tsp sunflower oil
2 small red onions, chopped
4 tsp tamari
1 tsp balsamic vinegar

Preheat the oven to 350°F. First, make the pumpkin purée. Toss the pumpkin chunks with the rosemary and sunflower oil, place into a roasting tray, and roast for 30 minutes. Remove from the oven and transfer the contents of the tray to a blender. Blitz till smooth and set aside.

Next, heat the water in a pan and add the bouillon powder and star anise. Once the bouillon has dissolved, take the stock off the heat and set aside.

Heat the sunflower oil in a pan on low to medium heat. Add the onions and garlic and gently sauté. Add the za'atar and the rice and stir everything around the pan for a minute or so. Then, slowly start adding the stock to the rice, around ⅓ cup at a time, stirring all the time. Once the rice has absorbed the liquid, feed it with more.

Meanwhile, start the onions. Heat the oil in a pan on low to medium heat. Add the onions and sauté. When translucent, add the balsamic and tamari, and sauté for 12 minutes; don't let them burn!

Once all the liquid has been absorbed, add the orange juice and the pumpkin purée to the risotto. Stir for another 5 minutes; if it looks too thick, add 1 to 2 tablespoons of water. Garnish and serve with a squeeze of lemon and the lovely soft onions.

NUTRITIONAL NUGGET
Pumpkin is full of beta-carotene—an important antioxidant that helps to ward off tummy bugs and protect the lining of the intestines.

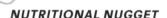

Mulled Wine
The benefits of antioxidants found in red wine over white are manifold. This warmed, spicy wine at Halloween (or indeed any other autumnal or winter events) can be nourishing and relaxing!

MAKES 4 SMALL OR 2 LARGE GLASSES
1 bottle of red wine (Chianti Classico is perfect)
juice of 1 orange and 1 lemon
4 star anise
1 cinnamon stick
5-6 cloves (optional—not everyone likes them)
1 orange, halved and sliced for visual effect!
Combine all the ingredients in a heavy-bottom pan and place over low heat, to allow the flavors to meld for at least 1 hour before serving. Double or quadruple the ingredients if you're having a party! Check the temperature on the back of a wooden spoon before serving, so as not to burn your lips. Serve warm, but not too hot.

SHREDDED MANGO, CARROT, AND CILANTRO SALAD

*If you've had enough of the sweet stuff that goes
hand-in-hand with trick or treating, then try this twist
on an Asian salad. It's crunchy, sweet, and tangy and
makes a perfect side dish or a main; and it's easy to
double up when friends are coming over. Serve with
a mixed leaf salad to boost the portion size.*

serves 2 as a salad or 4 as a side dish

2 carrots

1 mango

¼ tsp black onion seeds

½ tsp raw sesame seeds

finely grated zest of 1 lime

3 tbsp cilantro, finely chopped

First, make the Sweet Chili Dipping Sauce as
instructed on page 82.

Peel and grate the carrots. Then, peel the mango
and cut it into thin slices.

Toast the black onion and sesame seeds by heating
them in a dry pan until the sesame seeds start to
change to a golden color.

Keep all the elements of the salad separate until
just before you want to serve it. Then, toss
everything together in a bowl, along with a couple
of tablespoons of the sweet chili dressing and serve
straightaway.

TASH'S TIPS

If you are serving this up at a dinner
party, dress it just before serving, as
the vegetables can easily wilt if done
too far in advance.

NUTRITIONAL NUGGET

Mango is rich in magnesium, a
mineral that is often deficient when
you're stressed and tired. So give
yourself a mango boost!

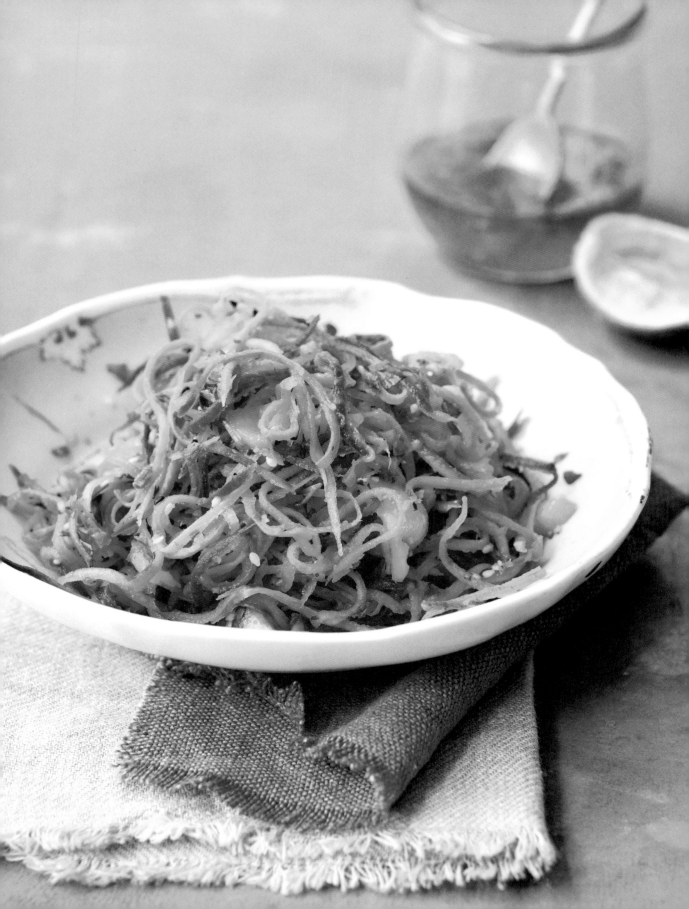

BIRTHDAY GET-TOGETHER

WHITE CHOCOLATE ROSE CUPS

Games will pause, conversations will halt, and mouths will hang open when you bring a tray of these stunning treats into the room. What's more, they freeze well, so make a big batch and keep a small stash in the freezer. Bring them out for an after-dinner treat anytime—the perfect "here's one I made earlier" dessert!

makes 24

For the filling:
½ cup dates, pitted
¼ cup raw pecans
1½ tbsp raw cacao powder

For the "white" chocolate:
scant ½ cup raw cashew nuts
scant 1 cup raw cacao butter
1 vanilla bean, split and scraped
1½ tbsp agave sugar
24 dried rose buds or petals (one per chocolate)

First, make the filling. Soak the dates for 30 minutes in warm water, then drain. Blend in a food processor with the pecans (you want small chunks of nut) and cacao powder. Set aside in a bowl while you make the "white" chocolate.

To make the "white" chocolate, soak the cashews for 30 minutes in water, then drain. Melt the raw cacao butter in a heatproof bowl over a pan of simmering water, or in a bain marie, along with the seeds from the vanilla bean, and then leave to cool for 10 minutes.

Put the melted cacao, cashews, and agave sugar in a high-speed blender and blitz until very smooth—you now have some "white" chocolate. (You will need a high-speed blender otherwise the cashews might be too chunky. If you don't have one, you could buy the same weight of white cashew butter and blend this with the cacao butter and agave sugar.)

In a silicone ice-cube tray or chocolate mold, pour enough of the chocolate mixture to cover the bottom of 24 molds; don't put too much in as you need to be able to fill them. Pop in the freezer for 15 minutes to set.

Remove from the freezer and add around ⅛ teaspoon of the filling into the center of the mold, then pour more white chocolate on top, so that it goes around the filling and over the top. Then, push a rose bud or petal into the top of each one and return to the freezer for 30 minutes to set.

Pop them out of the molds and enjoy watching your guests demolish them.

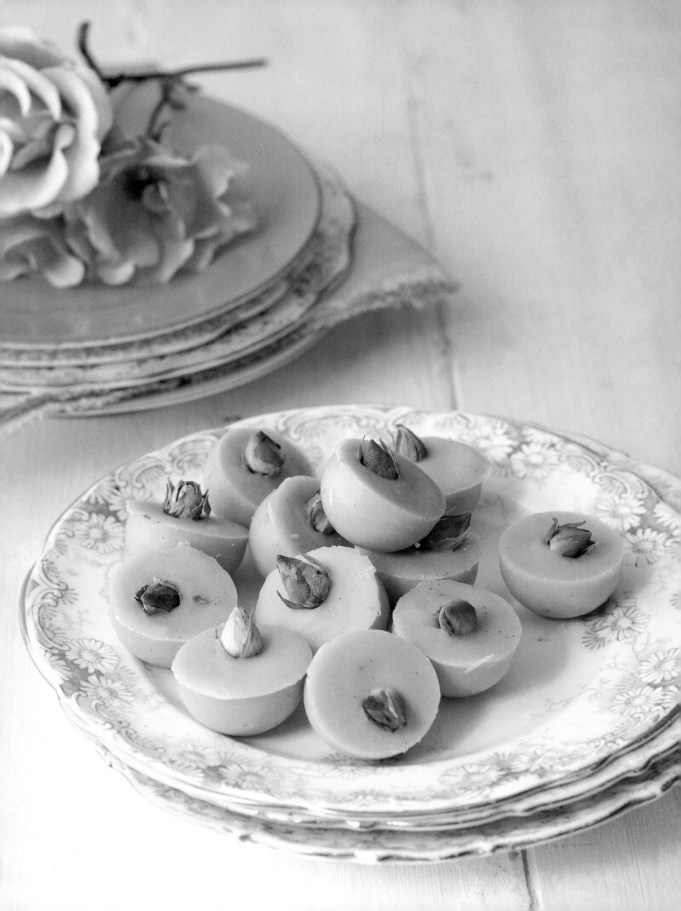

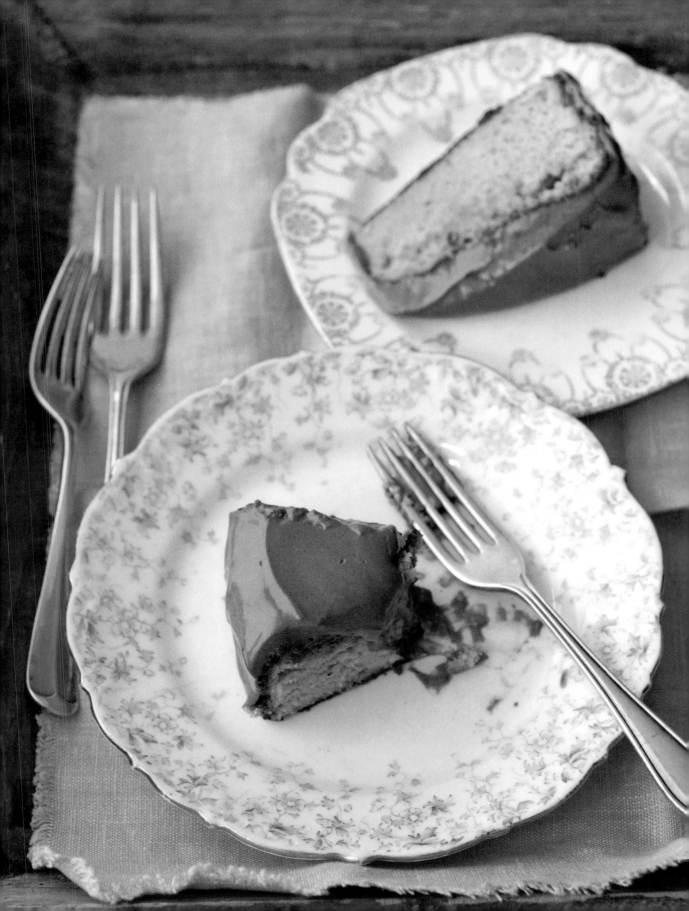

ORANGE AND ALMOND CAKE WITH ORANGE SYRUP AND CHOCOLATE FROSTING

This light and airy cake is one of the simplest cakes to bake and makes a great birthday cake. If you're after a less indulgent version, then simply opt for the one with vanilla cream (see right) rather than this glorious chocolate version.

serves 8

For the cake:
6 eggs
½ cup brown rice syrup or agave syrup
finely grated zest of 3 large oranges
1⅔ cups ground almonds

For the orange syrup:
juice of 3 large oranges
3 tbsp xylitol or brown rice syrup

For the chocolate frosting:
2 cups tofu cream cheese
½ cup agave syrup
5 tbsp raw cacao powder

Preheat the oven to 325°F, and grease and line a 9-inch springform cake pan with either vegan butter or sunflower oil.

Separate the eggs and put the whites into one large bowl and the yolks into another. Beat the yolks well, adding the syrup followed by the orange zest and ground almonds. Mix to combine well.

In a separate bowl, whisk the egg whites to stiff peaks. Then fold gently into the eggy orange mixture. Pour the batter into the prepared pan (the batter will be runny) and bake in the preheated oven for 40 minutes. Do keep checking the color of the top of your cake; if it starts to go brown too soon, cover with foil to stop the top from burning.

While the cake is baking, make the syrup. Simply heat the ingredients in a pan over medium heat until a thick syrup forms and set aside.

Take the cake out of the oven and prick all over with a toothpick, then pour over most of the orangey syrup while the cake is warm—keep some back and let it cool, use this for the final glaze.

While the cake is cooling on a wire rack, make the chocolate frosting. Beat the tofu cream cheese in a bowl with a spatula, add the agave and cacao, and continue to beat until mixed in and smooth. Add a final orange syrup glaze, then spread the frosting all over your cake, and slice and serve.

VARIATION Orange and almond cake with orange syrup and vanilla almond cream

For the vanilla almond cream:
1½ cups blanched almonds
1 cup water
½ vanilla bean, split and scraped, or
 ½ tsp vanilla extract
1 tsp brown rice syrup

Before you start the recipe (left), soak the almonds in water for 1 hour and set aside.

Make the recipe, on the left, up to and including pricking the cake and pouring on the syrup.

While the cake is cooling, drain the almonds from their soaking water and pop into a blender with the measured water. Blend until smooth, then add the vanilla seeds or extract with the rice syrup and blend again.

Serve a dollop of the vanilla-scented almond cream with a slice of the cake.

MANGO AND COCONUT RAW CHEESECAKE

*This is a healthy sweet treat that still feels indulgent.
It works well with other flavors, too; try substituting
the mango for the same weight of raspberries—it
will be beautiful and pink.*

serves 8

For the base:
generous 1 cup ground almonds
¼ tsp Himalayan pink salt
½ cup medjool dates, pitted and chopped
  finely
½ tsp finely grated lime zest
½ tsp ground ginger

For the filling:
1½ cups raw cashew nuts
1 tbsp finely grated lime zest (around 1½ limes)
scant ¼ cup lime juice
scant ¼ cup coconut oil, melted
⅓ cup coconut water
2 tbsp vanilla extract (or seeds scraped from
  2 vanilla beans)
½ tsp yeast flakes
1 large very ripe mango (around 9 oz), sliced

For the topping:
1 small mango, sliced
fresh coconut, grated, or dry unsweetened
  coconut

Line an 8-inch cake pan with plastic wrap. Cover
the raw cashews with water and soak for 30
minutes, then drain.

In a bowl, mix the ground almonds and salt
together. Using your hands, mix in the dates, lime
zest, and ginger, squeezing to form a dough. Rub
the mixture through your fingers until it reaches a
bread crumb-like consistency.

Sprinkle over the bottom of the cake pan,
sprinkling more thickly at the sides. Then press
the crumbs onto the base and up the sides until you
have your cheesecake crust.

To make the filling, blend all the ingredients
together until smooth and creamy. Pour the filling
on top evenly and place in the refrigerator to set,
for at least 3 to 4 hours or ideally overnight.

Before serving, top with some vibrant slices of
mango and grate some fresh coconut or sprinkle
dry unsweetened coconut over it, if you prefer.

TASH'S TIPS

If you are going to try a new flavor—
here's another winning formula. Use
cinnamon in the base instead of
ginger, remove the lime, and go for
fresh cherries on the top.

NUTRITIONAL NUGGET

Cashew nuts are rich in the minerals
zinc and selenium (great for
immunity), as well as having high
levels of oleic acid and other
monounsaturated fats, which help to
redress the types of cholesterol in
your blood to a much more healthy
balance.

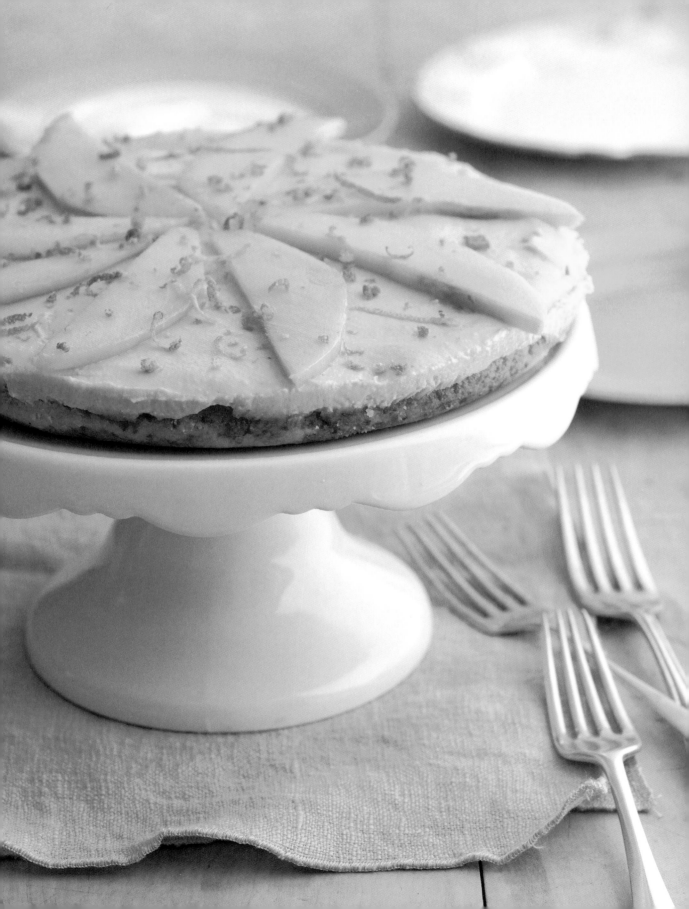

EASTER

RAW CHOCOLATE EGGS

The perfect fix for any chocoholic! Enjoy experimenting with mold shapes—we love eggs at this time of year—and with different flavors. A little drop of peppermint, orange, or ginger extract can make a world of difference to the taste. Of course, chocolate is not only for Easter—you can use this recipe year round whenever you want an intense and chocolatey treat.

makes 24

1 cup raw cacao butter

¾ cup raw cacao powder

⅓ cup agave syrup

½ tsp vanilla extract

1 drop of flavored extract (optional)

Melt the raw cacao butter in a heatproof bowl over a pan of simmering water or in a bain marie. Allow it to cool for around 10 minutes, then add the cacao powder and mix in. Once incorporated, add the agave, vanilla, and flavored extract, if using.

Pour the chocolate into whatever silicone molds you're using and put straight into the freezer for 30 minutes, or until set.

Pop them out and keep in the refrigerator. Serve chilled.

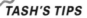

TASH'S TIPS
If you want to color layers of your chocolate or speckle the eggs just do one layer of color, put back into the freezer to set for 20 minutes, then layer with another color and repeat the freezing until you're happy with the result.

NUTRITIONAL NUGGET
Raw cacao has one of the highest sources of vitamin K, which is essential for the absorption of calcium into your bones.

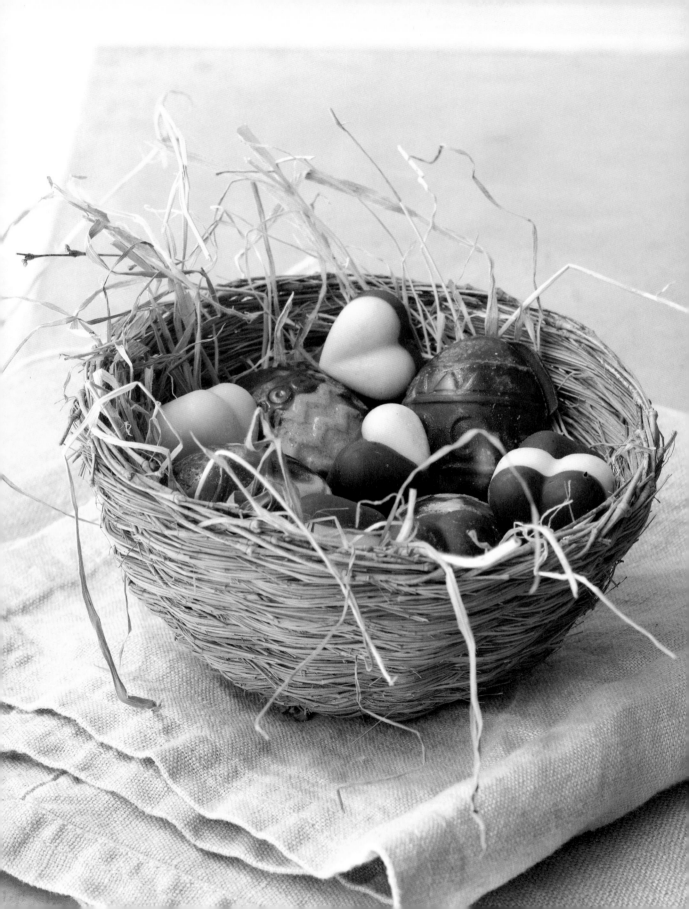

SPINACH PANCAKES WITH CARROT PURÉE

This wonderfully light dish just sings of springtime, with its vibrant colors and super-nutritious content. Why not try it out on some guests over the Easter holiday weekend and see what they make of it? Either serve them already rolled up or let people just help themselves—it's up to you.

makes 4 to 6 pancakes

For the pancakes:

3 oz spinach

½ clove garlic

generous ½ cup buckwheat flour

scant ½ cup rice flour

1 tsp baking powder

½ tsp Himalayan pink salt

1 egg, beaten

1⅔ cups brown rice milk

1 tbsp lemon juice

1 tbsp sunflower oil, plus extra for greasing

2 tbsp rice syrup

For the purée:

4 large carrots, boiled until soft, then drained well

2 tbsp olive oil

a handful of flat-leaf parsley

a pinch of Himalayan pink salt

Put the spinach and garlic into a blender and pulse until you have a rough purée.

Place the buckwheat flour, rice flour, baking powder, and salt in a large bowl and mix well.

Place the egg, milk, lemon juice, sunflower oil, and rice syrup in another bowl and mix well, then stir into the dry ingredients and mix gently until just combined, being careful not to overmix.

Wipe a skillet lightly with oil and heat over medium heat. Place a poachette ring or pastry ring in the pan and ladle in 1 tablespoon of the pancake batter. Cook until air bubbles start to appear on the surface of the pancake. Do not turn until this point. Remove the mold, turn the pancake, and cook for around 1 minute on the other side, until set. Repeat until all the batter is used and cooked.

Blend the carrots, oil, a handful of parsley, and the salt until smooth. Serve this carrot purée with the pancakes and some salad leaves or just as an accompaniment to a delicious salad.

NUTRITIONAL NUGGET

Buckwheat contains rutin—a compound associated with strengthening capillary walls all over the brain and body.

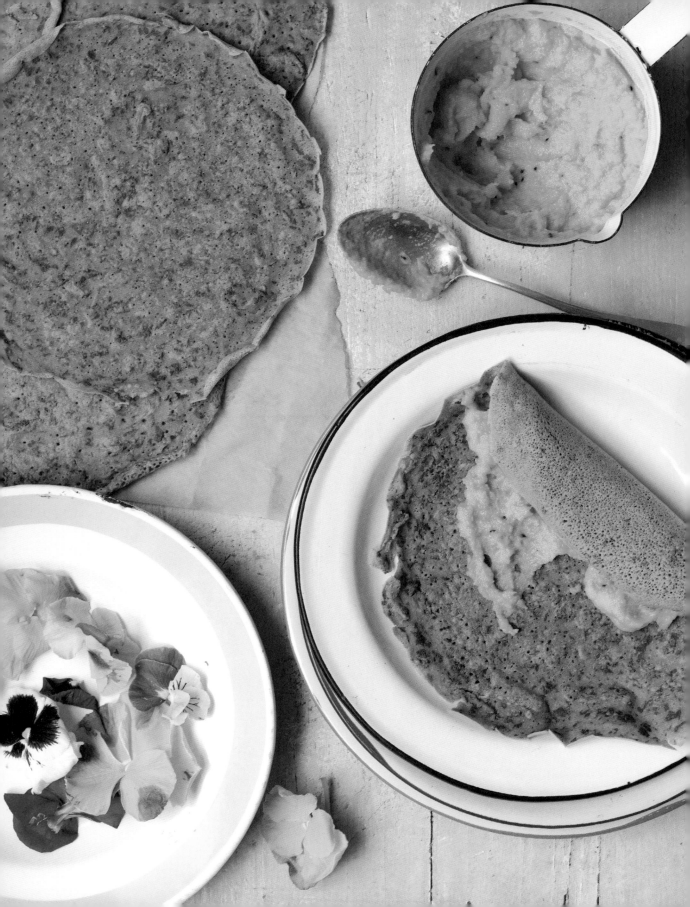

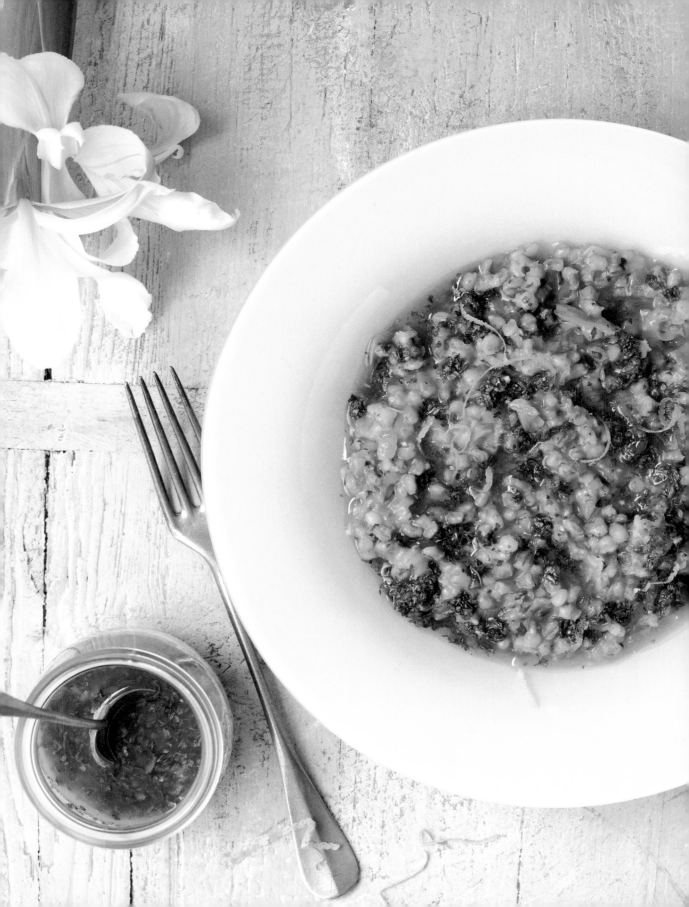

LEMON "RISOTTO"

If you've overindulged on chocolate eggs, then reach for this zesty "risotto." It's really easy to make and once you've tried out this lemon version, you can experiment with other flavors as your whim takes you—I love leek and fennel, for instance.

♥ ♥ ♥

serves 2

1 tbsp bouillon powder

3¾ cups boiling water

1 tbsp sunflower oil

½ red onion, chopped

1 clove garlic, chopped

finely grated zest of 2 lemons, plus extra to garnish

juice of 2 lemons

½ cup pearl barley

1 bay leaf

For the parsley oil:

½ cup olive oil

1¼ oz flat-leaf parsley

a pinch of salt

finely grated zest and juice of 1 lemon

Add the bouillon powder to the boiling water to make a vegetable stock and stir until all the powder has dissolved. Set aside.

Heat the sunflower oil in a pan on medium heat. Add the onions and garlic and sauté together for 1 to 2 minutes. Then add scant ¼ cup of the stock to the pan. When that water has become a thicker sauce with the onions, add another scant ¼ cup of stock along with half the lemon zest and all of the lemon juice.

Add the pearl barley and bay leaf to the pan and ladle in the remaining stock as the barley absorbs it. Keep adding the stock and stirring until it is absorbed—this will take around 20 minutes. The trick is to stir the pearl barley continuously to make it creamy without adding any dairy products. Once it's ready, add the remaining lemon zest and remove the bay leaf.

To make the parsley oil, simply blend all of the ingredients together for 30 seconds.

Then take the pan off the heat and serve with a drizzle of parsley oil over the top and a little zest.

TASH'S TIPS

If you like to super-charge the lemon here, just increase the quantity of lemons juiced. However citrusy you like your flavors, be sure to stir, stir, stir so the "risotto" is really creamy.

NUTRITIONAL NUGGET

Pearl barley, a seemingly old-fashioned but nutrient-dense grain, is packed with beta-glucan, known to lower cholesterol and balance blood sugar levels. It is an excellent long-lasting energy food.

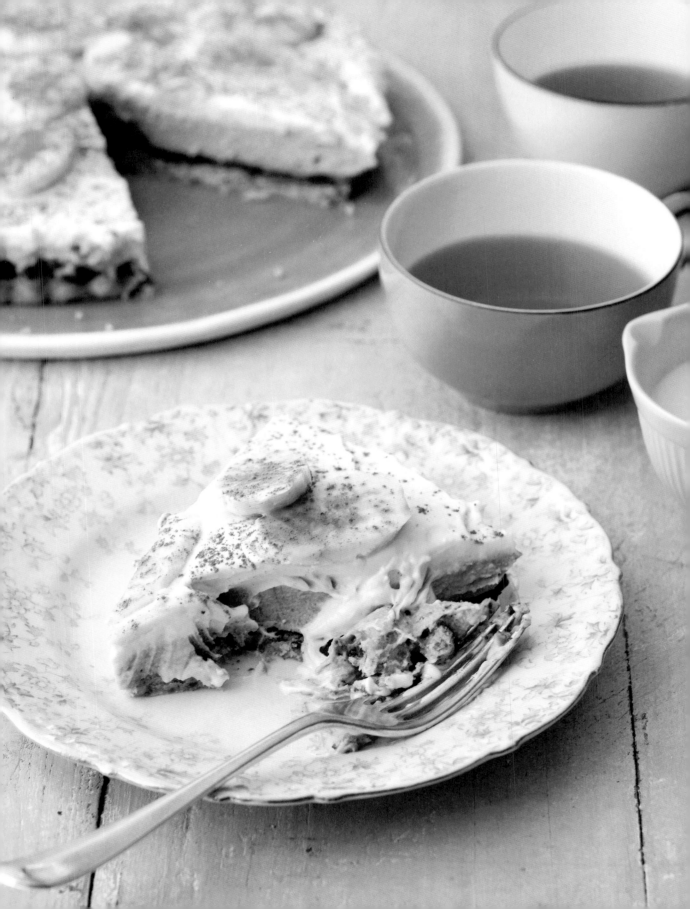

RAW BANOFFEE PIE

To me, banoffee pie equals Easter. At school this was my favorite dessert. My friend's mother made the best one and the secret was a hidden layer of chocolate. We always looked forward to her birthday, so we could get our banoffee fix. I have always wanted to try to make a healthier version and here it is!

serves 10

For the base:
1⅔ cups ground almonds
⅓ cup raw almonds
3½ oz dates
2 tbsp coconut oil

For the chocolate sauce:
3 tbsp coconut oil
2 tbsp raw cacao powder
2 tbsp date syrup

For the filling:
scant 1 cup raw cashew nuts
generous ½ cup sugar-free almond milk
⅛ tsp vanilla extract
3 large ripe bananas
3 tbsp coconut palm sugar
1 tbsp date syrup

For the dairy-free cream:
8 tbsp tofu cream cheese, at room temperature
8 tbsp vegan butter, at room temperature
4 tbsp agave syrup or powdered agave
½ tsp vanilla extract

First, make the base. Put all the ingredients into a food processor and blitz until the almonds and dates are small chunks—when you squeeze it together in your hands it will stick together.

Line an 8½-inch tart pan with plastic wrap; if you don't have a tart pan, a cake pan will do.

Tip the mixture from the processor into the pan and press down into the bottom so that it's packed tightly. Put into the freezer for 30 minutes to set.

Cover the raw cashews with cold water and soak for 30 minutes.

Meanwhile, make the chocolate sauce by melting the coconut oil in a heatproof bowl over a pan of simmering water or in a bain marie. Add the cacao powder and date syrup, mix well, and then leave to cool in the bowl.

Drain the soaked cashews and put into a high-speed blender along with the almond milk, vanilla, 2 of the bananas, palm sugar, and date syrup. Blend until very smooth.

Take the base out of the freezer and pour the chocolate sauce over the top. Next, pour over the filling and return to the freezer for 1 hour, until set.

Next, make the dairy-free cream. Put all the ingredients into a bowl and mix together (I use the back of a wooden spoon) until you have a smooth, creamy consistency, then set aside in the refrigerator. It'll thicken up while it's setting.

Slice the remaining banana and take the pie out of the freezer. You can either arrange the banana over the top, then serve with the cream on the side or spread on the cream as the uppermost layer and then place the banana slices on top.

Remove the pie from its pan just before serving and dust with a little raw cacao powder.

MUMMY'S BAKED APPLES

This is my mother's staple dessert whenever we go over for a Sunday lunch and that means at Easter, too. But it's a great healthy finish to any meal. I always joke with her that this is the only thing she can cook, but it's so delicious I have borrowed it for the book with a few extra tweaks. Enjoy!

makes 6

6 cooking apples

6 dates

1 cup mixed-color raisins

⅓ cup agave syrup

juice of 1 orange

3 star anise

cold water

½ tbsp cinnamon

finely grated zest of 1 orange

Preheat the oven to 350°F. You'll need an ovenproof baking sheet.

Core the apples and place them on the baking sheet. Push a date into each of the apple's cores and stuff the rest of the hole with the raisins—sprinkle the rest of the raisins around into the dish. Drizzle the agave syrup evenly over the top of the apples and then also into the bottom of the dish. Pour in the orange juice and pop the star anise in.

Pour in cold water so that it fills the dish to ½-inch up the sides. Then sprinkle the cinnamon and orange zest over the apples and into the water; the water is going to create a lovely syrup.

Bake in the preheated oven for 40 to 45 minutes, until the apples burst and go crispy on the outside. I like them bursting, but if you don't want them to burst, cut a small line around ⅛-inch thick around the "equator" of the apple before baking.

Serve with the juices from the dish or with a dollop of yogurt.

TASH'S TIPS

If you want to try out a less traditional flavor, then use a combination of goji berries and dry unsweetened coconut instead of the dates and raisins for a fab taste.

NUTRITIONAL NUGGET

Apples contain pectin, which helps remove toxins from the digestive system, as well as feeds the beneficial bacteria that live there.

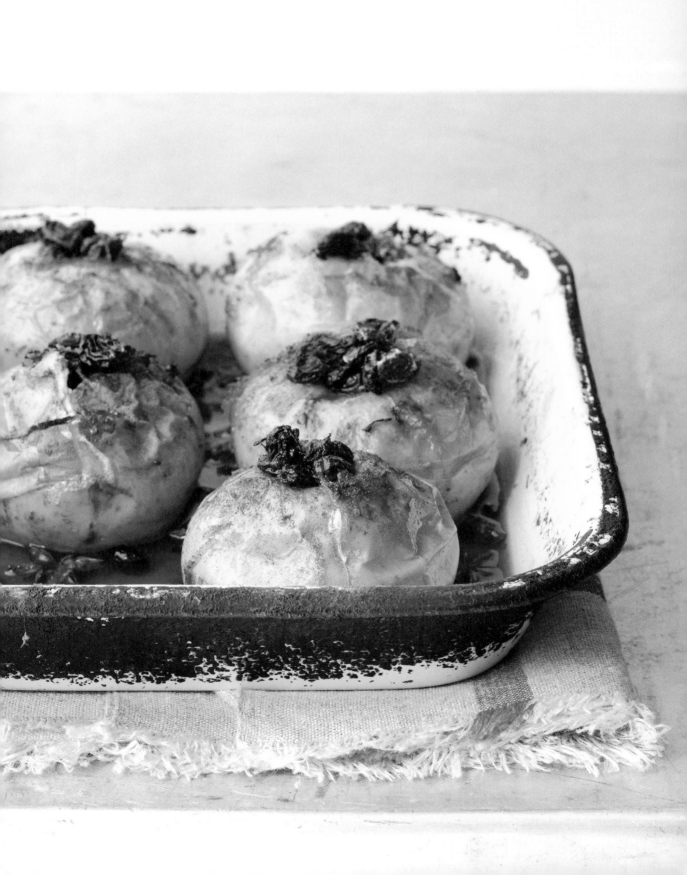

HERE COME THE HOLIDAYS

BEJEWELED BRUSSELS SPROUTS

Brussels sprouts have such bad press, but I love them. They are especially delicious when roasted and work perfectly with the added sweetness of the cranberries. I am sure you can persuade even the biggest Brussels sprout cynic that this is the new dish to eat!

serves 6 as a side dish

1 lb 10 oz Brussels sprouts

6 cloves of garlic, with skin still on

2 tbsp sunflower oil

⅛ tsp Himalayan pink salt

cracked black pepper

scant 1 cup unsweetened dried cranberries

½ cup flat-leaf parsley, chopped

1 tbsp mirin

Preheat the oven to 325°F. You'll need a baking sheet.

Trim the brown ends off the Brussels sprouts, pull off any yellow outer leaves, and cut the sprouts in half. In a bowl, mix them with the garlic cloves, sunflower oil, salt, and pepper.

Transfer to the baking sheet and roast in the preheated oven for 35 to 40 minutes, until crisp on the outside and tender on the inside. Shake the tray from time to time to brown the sprouts evenly.

Meanwhile, soak the cranberries in water for 30 minutes then drain and set aside.

Remove the Brussels sprouts from the oven and mix together with the parsley, mirin, and cranberries and serve immediately. These also work well stirred through cooked quinoa or added to a leafy salad.

TASH'S TIPS
Brussels sprouts are not just for Christmas—this dish works well added to a luscious salad with our Tahini Dressing (see page 82).

NUTRITIONAL NUGGET
Brussels sprouts have the highest levels of the cancer-protective glucosinolates of all the cruciferous vegetables. Tuck in!

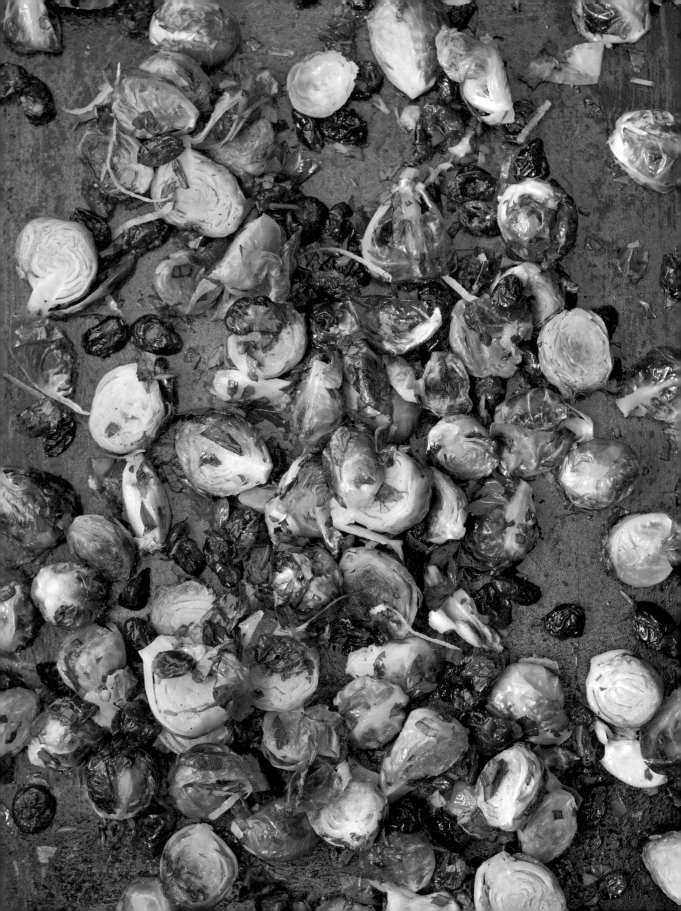

MY PUMPKIN PIE

I have always been intrigued by pumpkin pie—it being both sweet and savory—so I had great fun creating this recipe.

serves 6 to 8

For the crust:
⅓ cup dates, pitted
¼ cup hot water
1 tbsp sunflower oil
2¼ cups ground almonds
⅛ tsp ground nutmeg

For the filling:
1 lb 5 oz pumpkin, peeled and roughly chopped
1 tbsp sunflower oil
3 eggs
1 tsp ground cinnamon
¼ tsp ground ginger
¼ tsp mixed spice
1 tsp vanilla extract
1 tbsp coconut flour
2 tbsp agave syrup

Preheat the oven to 325°F, and line a 6-inch tart pan with parchment paper.

Soak the dates for 10 minutes in the measured water, then drain.

Put all the crust ingredients into a food processor and pulse until they come together to form a ball. Carefully tip the ball into the pan and press the "dough" evenly all around.

Prick the dough and bake for 15 to 20 minutes, or until lightly golden. Remove from the oven and let cool for 20 minutes before adding the filling.

Roast the pumpkin with the sunflower oil for 20 minutes until it is soft. Remove from the oven and let cool.

Transfer the roasted pumpkin to a blender and whiz until smooth. Then add the eggs, spices, vanilla extract, coconut flour, and agave syrup and blend again until you get a super-smooth mixture. Scoop the mixture up and transfer into the crust and bake for 30 to 40 minutes. Remove from the oven and let cool.

No need for any accompaniments, it's delicious just on its own.

TASH'S TIPS
Make sure you allow the pumpkin to cool after it has come out of the oven and before you put the eggs in as you don't want them to scramble.

NUTRITIONAL NUGGET
Pumpkin is packed with zeaxanthin, an antioxidant that helps to protect the eyes from age-related degeneration.

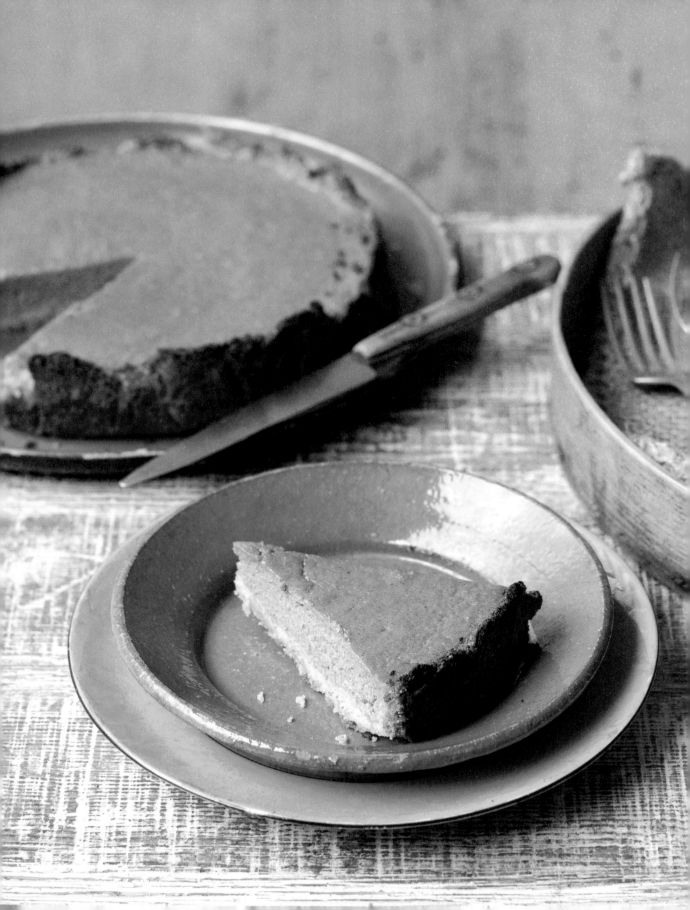

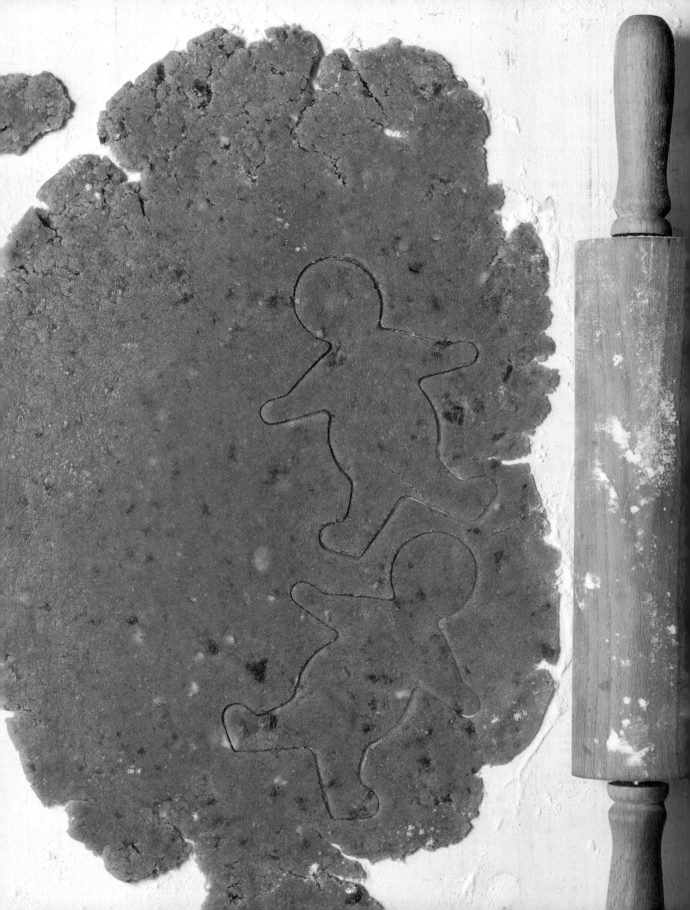

GINGERBREAD MEN

*If the smell of these baking doesn't transport you
back to childhood, the taste of them surely will.
These are one of the easiest recipes to make—in
fact, perfect for little helpers—and make delicious
Christmas tree decorations, too.*

makes 8

For the cookies:

3 cups ground almonds

1 tsp ground cinnamon

½ tsp ground ginger

¼ tsp ground nutmeg

½ tsp baking powder

6 dates, pitted

3 tbsp coconut oil, melted

5 tbsp rice syrup

1 tsp vanilla extract

1 egg white

For the frosting:

⅓ cup coconut milk

½ cup rice or almond milk powder

4 tbsp agave syrup

1 tsp vanilla extract

⅔ cup coconut oil, melted

1 tbsp lemon juice

Put the almonds, spices, baking powder, and dates
into a food processor and pulse. Add the coconut
oil, rice syrup, vanilla extract, and egg white and
pulse again until everything comes together to
form a ball of dough. Transfer the gingerbread
dough to a bowl, cover it with plastic wrap, and chill
for 1 hour.

Preheat the oven to 325°F and line a baking sheet
with parchment paper.

Roll out the chilled gingerbread to a thickness of
⅛ inch, and then, using a cookie cutter, cut out little
men (or any other shape you fancy) and place them
on the prepared baking sheet.

Bake in the preheated oven for 20 minutes.
Remove from the oven and let cool on a wire rack.

Next, make the frosting by putting all the
ingredients, apart from the coconut oil and lemon
juice, in a food processor or blender and whiz until
smooth. Then add the coconut oil and lemon juice
and blend again until combined and silky smooth.
Transfer the frosting to a pastry bag and chill for 2
hours; the longer in the refrigerator the better, so
that the frosting isn't too runny and then it's easy to
draw on cute little faces.

When the gingerbread cookies are completely cool,
decorate them however you like—I like to pipe
faces and clothes onto our gingerbread men.

NUTRITIONAL NUGGET
Coconut oil and coconut milk are rich
in medium-chain-fats, which help
ease digestive complaints and lower
the development of type 2 diabetes.
Eat a teaspoon every day.

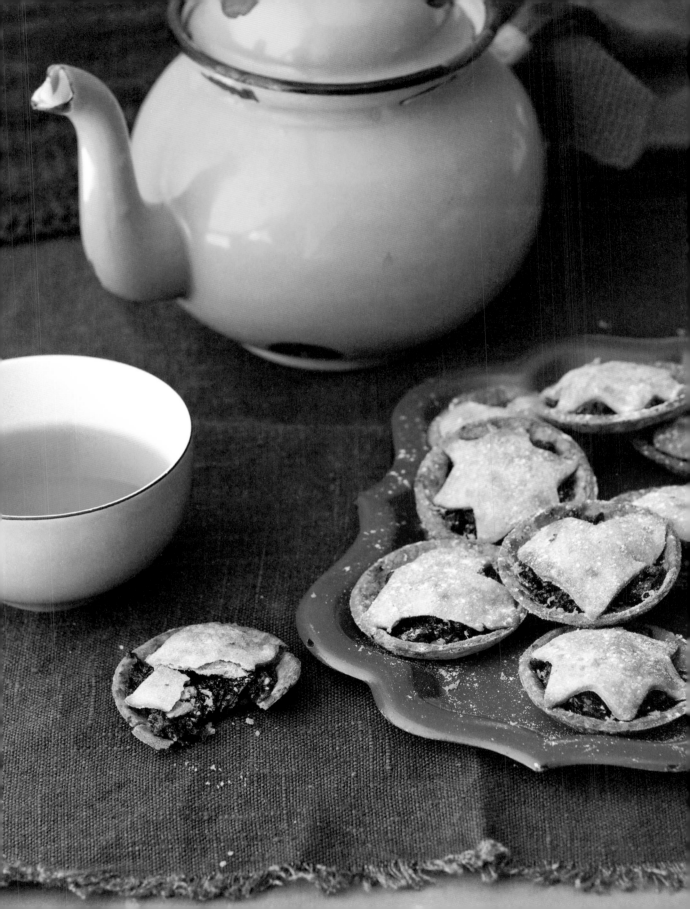

MINCEMEAT PIES

*Christmas wouldn't be Christmas without
mincemeat pies, so I had to find a way of making a
healthy version to keep up with tradition. I think I've
found a tastier option—try them and see for yourself.*

makes 12

For the pastry:
4 tbsp vegan butter, plus extra for greasing
4 tbsp coconut palm sugar
½ tsp vanilla extract
½ cup rice flour, plus extra for dusting
½ cup chickpea flour (gram)
scant ½ cup cornstarch
¼ tsp xanthan gum
a pinch of Himalayan pink salt
3 tsp water

For the filling:
scant ½ cup unsweetened dried blueberries
⅔ cup unsweetened dried cranberries
scant ½ cup golden raisins
finely grated zest of 1 orange
juice of ½ orange
finely grated zest of 1 lemon
¼ tsp grated nutmeg
1 tsp ground cinnamon

First, make the pastry. In a bowl, cream together
the butter, sugar, and vanilla extract. In a separate
bowl, mix together the flours, xanthan gum, and
salt. Pour the flour mix into the butter mixture,
add the water, and use your fingers to mix it
together to form a dough. Knead for a minute,
then roll into a ball, wrap in plastic wrap, and chill
for 30 minutes.

Meanwhile, put all the ingredients for the filling in
a food processor and pulse until you achieve a
rough consistency.

Preheat the oven to 325°F, and grease a 12-hole
muffin pan with vegan butter.

Dust a counter with some rice flour and roll out
the pastry to a thickness of ⅛ inch. Using a cookie
cutter, stamp out 12 circles, rerolling the
trimmings and cutting again; keep the remaining
pastry aside. Use these circles to line the base and
sides of each muffin "hole".

Fill each pie with 1 tablespoon of the mincemeat —
don't overfill or it will bubble out during cooking.

With the remaining pastry, roll out to a thickness of
⅛ inch and, using a shaped cutter (I like to use a
heart or a star), cut out 12 shapes that will form
your pie lids. Place over the filling, pushing the
edges of the lids down to meet the bottom pastry
rim. Bake in a preheated oven for 10 to 15 minutes.

Remove from the oven, leave to cool, and then
transfer to a wire rack. Dust with some rice flour or
agave powder and enjoy while still warm.

NUTRITIONAL NUGGET
Blueberries and cranberries are rich
in iron, fiber, and beta-carotene to
boost your immunity and give you
natural energy.

GLUTEN-FREE BREAD AND BUTTER PUDDING

In my family, this is our pudding of choice at Christmas. This recipe has to be dedicated to my mother: growing up she wasn't allowed bread and as a kid she loved this dessert...the secret is that this version is probably better than the real thing!

serves 6

4 cups almond milk

2 tsp vanilla extract

2 tbsp agave syrup

4 eggs

2 tbsp cornstarch

a pinch of ground nutmeg

10½ oz gluten-free bread

1½ tbsp vegan butter

⅔ cup raisins

Heat the almond milk in a pan over medium to high heat, with the vanilla extract and agave, and bring it to almost boiling point, then take off the heat.

Beat the eggs with the cornstarch and nutmeg in a mixing bowl until combined. Pour the hot milk over the eggs and whisk well. Pour the egg mixture back into the pan and cook over gentle heat, stirring with a wooden spoon in a figure-eight motion until the custard thickens and coats the back of the spoon.

Remove the custard from the heat, split it in half (keep half the custard for serving with the pudding later), and put a layer of plastic wrap over the top so that it does not develop a skin.

Grease and line a 9½ x 5½-inch loaf pan with parchment paper or, if you prefer, use an ovenproof dish of a similar size.

Cut your bread diagonally in half—so one slice will give you two triangles. Butter one side of each triangle of bread and, with the buttered-side-up, start building a layer of bread in the prepared pan, with a good scattering of raisins over each layer. Repeat the layers until you've used all the bread and raisins.

Pour one half of the custard over the bread. Let it stand for 30 minutes before baking. Preheat the oven to 325°F.

Bake in the preheated oven for 25 minutes. Remove from the oven and let cool a while.

Gently reheat the rest of the custard in a pan and serve while the pudding is warm.

NUTRITIONAL NUGGET

Cornstarch is relatively high in protein and helps to lower cholesterol owing to its fiber content. It is a good alternative to wheat for baking.

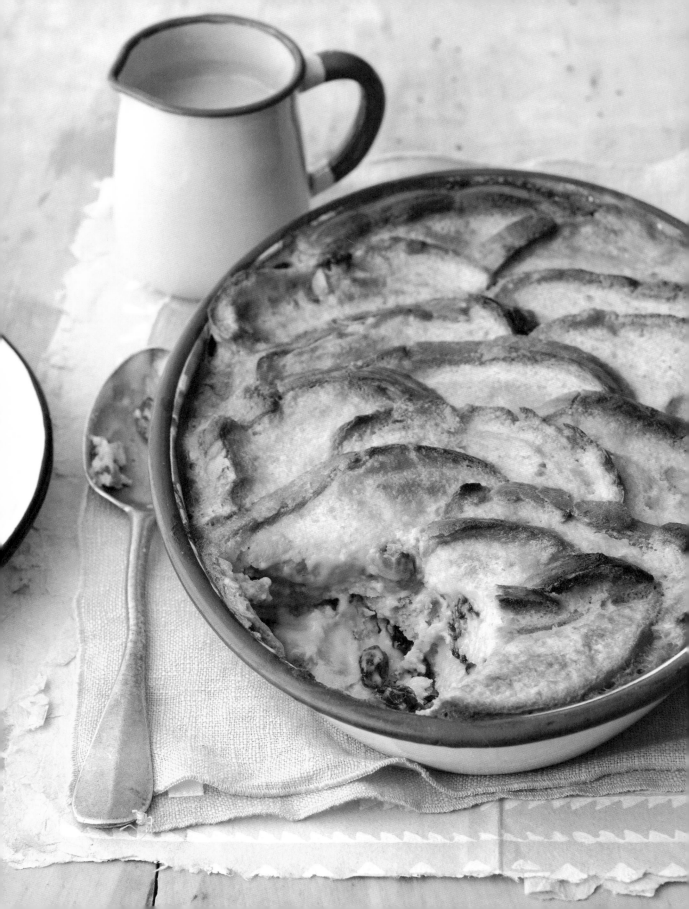

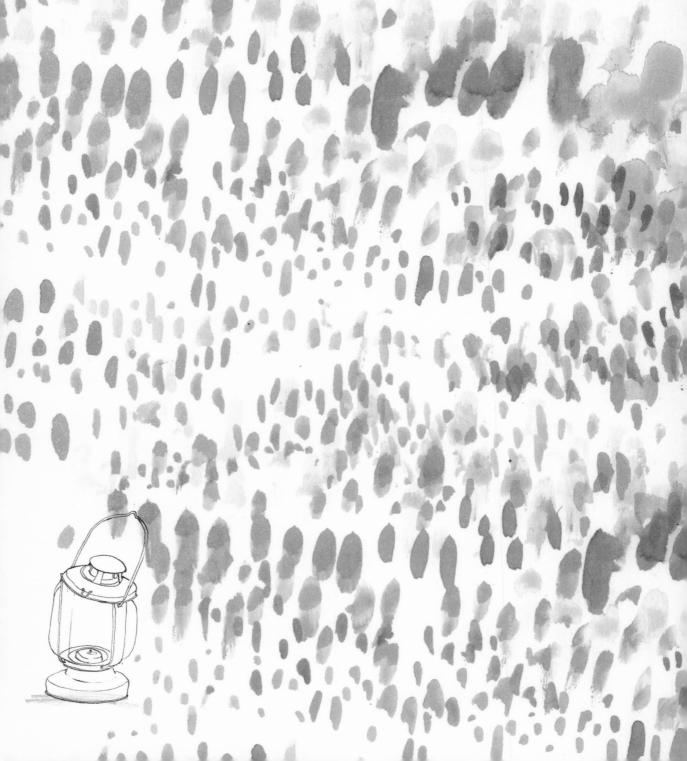

A BREATH

OF FRESH AIR

There is nothing better than being in the open air, especially when it comes to entertaining. I live in the UK where we are not blessed with consistently sunny warm days, so when they grace us with their presence I tend to run for the greenery. I love going for a picnic or having a BBQ with friends and family, especially when you can surprise them with your healthy vegetarian cooking skills and they don't even notice they are missing the traditional meaty options!

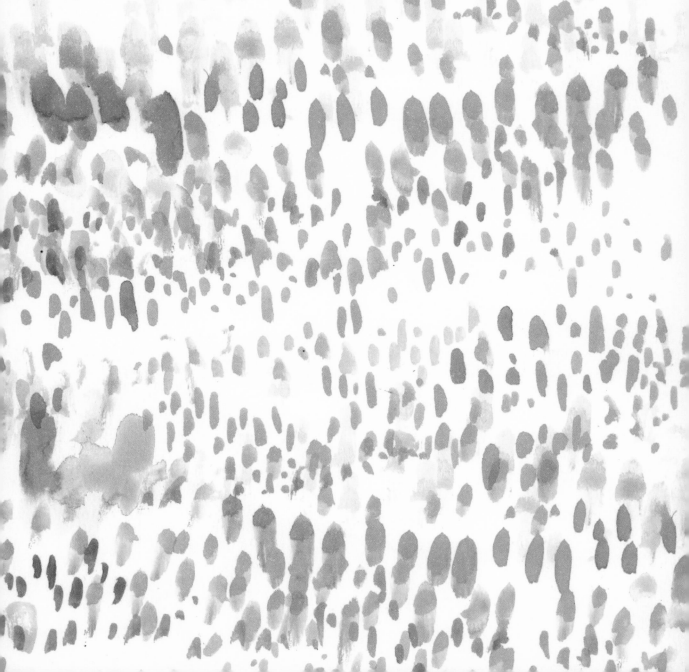

BARBECUE

PEPPERED TOFU BBQ SKEWERS

These BBQ delights could fool even the most hard-core of meat-eaters into thinking that tofu is the better alternative! If the weather's not right for cooking outside, then you can still enjoy these delicious skewers year round griddled or baked.

makes 6 skewers

4 oz tofu

1 tbsp sesame oil

1 tsp rice vinegar

5 tsp mixed peppercorns

1 tsp ground coriander

½ oz flat-leaf parsley

1 tsp grated or minced fresh ginger

1 tsp ground turmeric

juice of ½ lemon

½ clove garlic, crushed

¼ tsp pomegranate molasses

¼ fresh chili, finely sliced (optional)

For the skewers:

1 zucchini, cut into ¾-in chunks

1 leek, cut into ½-in chunks

1 red onion, cut into 6 or 8 segments

6 button or shiitake mushrooms

To serve:

6 scallions, griddled

6 mushrooms, griddled

Cut the tofu into ½-inch cubes and pop in a bowl with a marinade of sesame oil and rice vinegar. Soak the wooden skewers (if using) in water.

In a pestle and mortar (or a spice grinder), grind the mixed peppercorns to a semi-fine powder. Mix in the other ingredients and chili, if you're using. Coat the marinated tofu in the spicy peppercorn paste then you're ready to assemble the skewers.

Skewer the tofu and vegetables, separating each piece of tofu with a vegetable. Once assembled, brush more of the paste over the top and pop onto the grill. If you don't have a grill (or rain stops play), a griddle pan works just as well or you can even bake them in the oven (at 350°F) for 20 to 25 minutes.

I like to serve these skewers with griddled scallions and mushrooms.

TASH'S TIPS
If you have time, marinate the tofu for as long as you can. The longer you marinate it for, the more intense the flavors will be.

NUTRITIONAL NUGGET
Tofu is one of the best vegetarian sources of calcium for bone-building, and nearly 10% of its weight is complete protein.

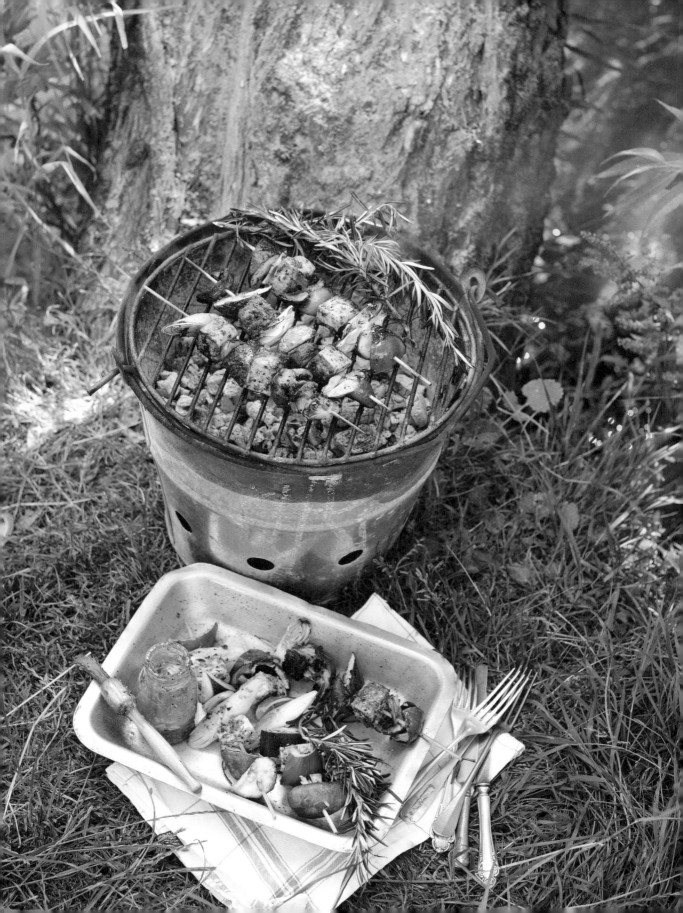

CORN ON THE COB

This is ridiculously easy to make, but so delicious and perfect for a BBQ, picnic, or garden party.

serves 4

4 corn on the cob
4 tbsp tamari
cracked black pepper

In a large pan, bring some water to a boil. Drop the corn into it when it's at a rolling boil and cook for 15 minutes. (If you want to pop it on the grill to finish it off, then boil for just 10 minutes and broil until golden.)

Take the cobs out of the water and place onto a plate. Drizzle with tamari and season with cracked pepper. And that's it!

NUTRITIONAL NUGGET
Corn on the cob provides one of the best sources of fiber, to ensure regular digestion, has anti-inflammatory powers, and is packed with vitamin C.

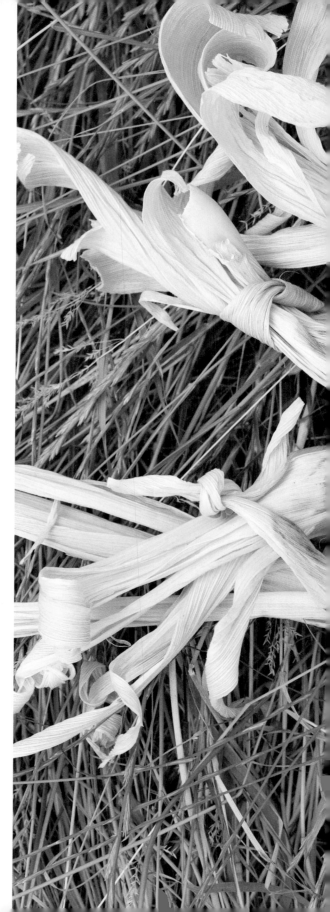

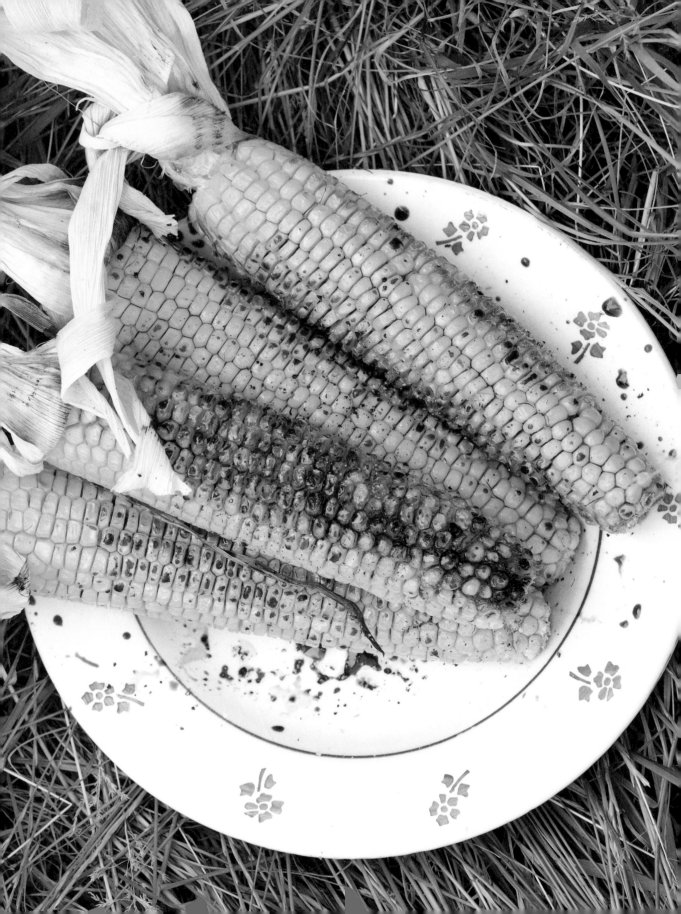

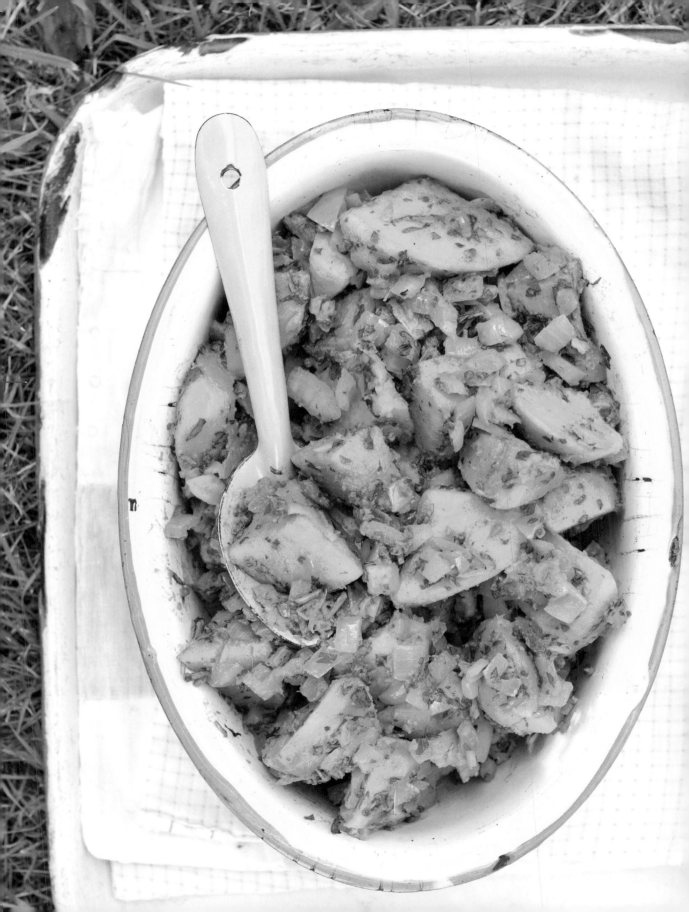

CURRIED SWEET POTATO

I love this great take on a traditional potato salad—and if you want to serve this as a main dish, then just add a few seeds or nuts on top and accompany with a gorgeous big leafy salad.

serves 6 as a side dish

1 large sweet potato (around 12 oz), cubed into
   1¼-in pieces
½ cup sunflower oil
2 tsp brown mustard seeds
2 tsp ground turmeric
2 tsp ground curry powder
2 tbsp finely minced ginger
2 tbsp finely minced garlic
½–1 tsp Celtic sea salt
2 white onions, finely chopped
⅓ cup cilantro, chopped
⅓ cup flat-leaf parsley, chopped

Lightly steam the sweet potato until tender (around 20 to 30 minutes) and set aside in a bowl. You don't want it too soft or it will become a mushy ball when mixed together.

Heat the oil in a wok on high heat and stir-fry the mustard seeds until they just pop. Next add the turmeric, curry powder, ginger, and garlic. Stir in the sea salt and onions and cook until the onions become translucent. Then, remove this curry paste from the heat.

Add the freshly chopped herbs and the curry paste to the sweet potato and stir until the sweet potato is uniformly coated with the mixture.

Serve with a green leaf salad.

Summer Breezer

There are those who simply cannot drink red wine, despite the health benefits, so this is a light Spritzer-style drink for the summer; the lime juice helps to alkalize an otherwise acid-forming drink.

MAKES 4 SMALL OR 2 LARGE GLASSES

6⅓ cups sparkling water
2 bottles of dry white wine
   (Sauvignon Blanc is ideal)
juice of 1 lime
lime slices, to decorate
mint leaves or rose petals, to decorate and add
   romance!

Mix the sparkling water, wine, and lime juice together. Serve in glasses with flowered ice cubes (see page 216) and lime slices. Decorate with mint leaves or rose petals, as you wish.

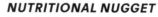

NUTRITIONAL NUGGET
Packed with vitamin C, beta-carotene, and magnesium, sweet potato has a lower glycemic index than its white alternatives, making it a great low-fat carbohydrate.

CARROT AND ZUCCHINI PATTIES

These are one of the simplest crowd pleasers to make, so much so that my friends actually request them now when they come for dinner. In my experience, kids love to eat them and help make them, especially squeezing the batter into patties. It's time to get your hands mucky!

makes 10

For the patties:
2 tbsp sunflower oil, plus 3–4 tbsp for frying
2 tbsp fennel seeds
4 large carrots, grated
1 zucchini, grated
4 scallions, chopped
1¼ oz cilantro, finely chopped
finely grated zest and juice of 1 lemon
generous ¾ cup halloumi, grated
1 clove garlic, crushed
2 tbsp red onion, grated
¼ cup rice flour
1 egg white

For the dressing:
4 tbsp olive oil
juice of 2 limes
1 tsp agave syrup
arugula leaves, to serve

Heat 2 tablespoons of oil in a pan over low heat and add the fennel seeds. Sauté for 3 minutes then take off the heat and set aside.

In a bowl, mix the remaining ingredients together along with the fennel seed oil.

Preheat the oven to 325°F. You'll need a baking sheet.

Take a handful of the mixture and squeeze out the moisture to make a small patty; it should fit in the palm of your hand. You'll probably be able to cook three or four patties at a time. For each batch, heat 1 tablespoon of oil in a skillet over medium heat. Sear each patty till golden on each side. Then bake on the sheet in the preheated oven for 15 minutes.

To make the dressing, simply mix all the ingredients together.

Remove the patties from the oven and serve three patties on a bed of arugula with the lime dressing drizzled over the top.

TASH'S TIPS
Make sure you squeeze out all the moisture when you are forming the patties, so they will stay together much better when you're sealing them.

NUTRITIONAL NUGGET
Zucchini are rich in potassium, zinc, and phosphorus, making them a superb mineral-rich, alkaline food.

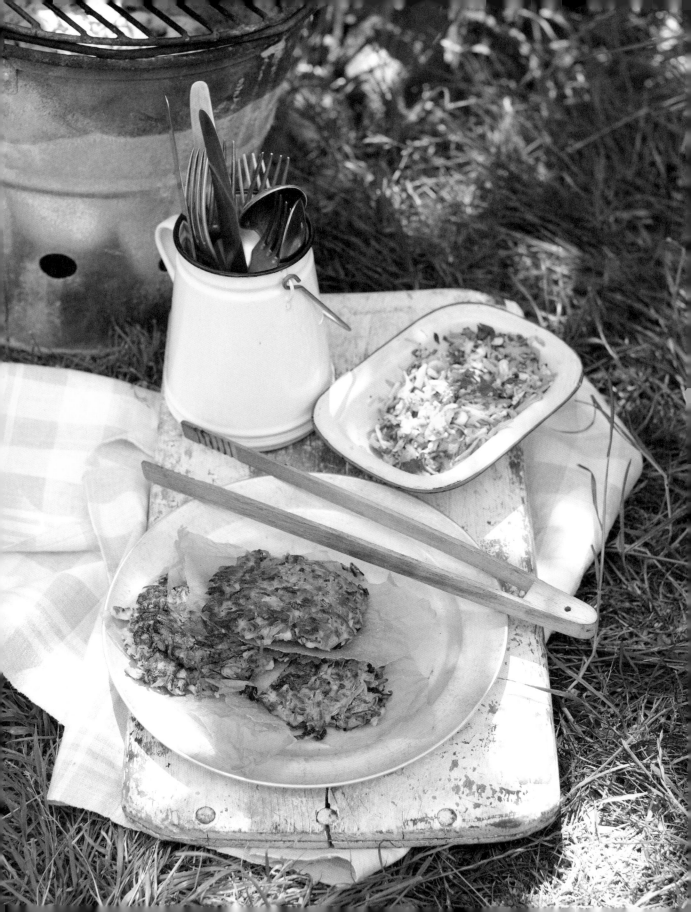

SPINACH AND CARROT MUFFINS

These are not your average muffins—when you make them, the batter looks more like it's going to be for patties, but when they're baked they are transformed into something truly divine.

makes 8

scant 1½ cups buckwheat flour

scant ¼ cup cornstarch

2 tsp baking powder

1 tsp xanthan gum

3 tbsp chia seeds, milled in a blender or spice grinder

½ tsp Himalayan pink salt

½ tsp nutmeg, grated

3 eggs

1 cup almond milk

7 oz fresh spinach leaves, roughly chopped

2 carrots (around 7 oz), grated

1 onion, grated

finely grated zest and juice of ½ lemon

1 clove garlic, grated

⅓ cup raw pumpkin seeds, for topping

Preheat the oven to 350°F. You'll need to line a 12-hole muffin pan with eight paper liners.

Mix the flours, baking powder, xanthan gum, chia seeds, salt, and nutmeg in a bowl and set aside.

Beat the eggs and almond milk together in another bowl. Add the spinach, carrots, onion, lemon zest and juice, and garlic. Stir for a minute and then pour in the dry ingredients. Mix gently to combine.

Pour the batter into the paper liners, top with the pumpkin seeds, and bake in a preheated oven for 25 minutes.

Remove the muffins from the oven, let cool in the pan for 20 minutes, then transfer to a wire rack to cool completely.

NUTRITIONAL NUGGET

Chia seeds contain the highest source of vegetarian omega-3 essential fats as well as abundant cholesterol-lowering fiber.

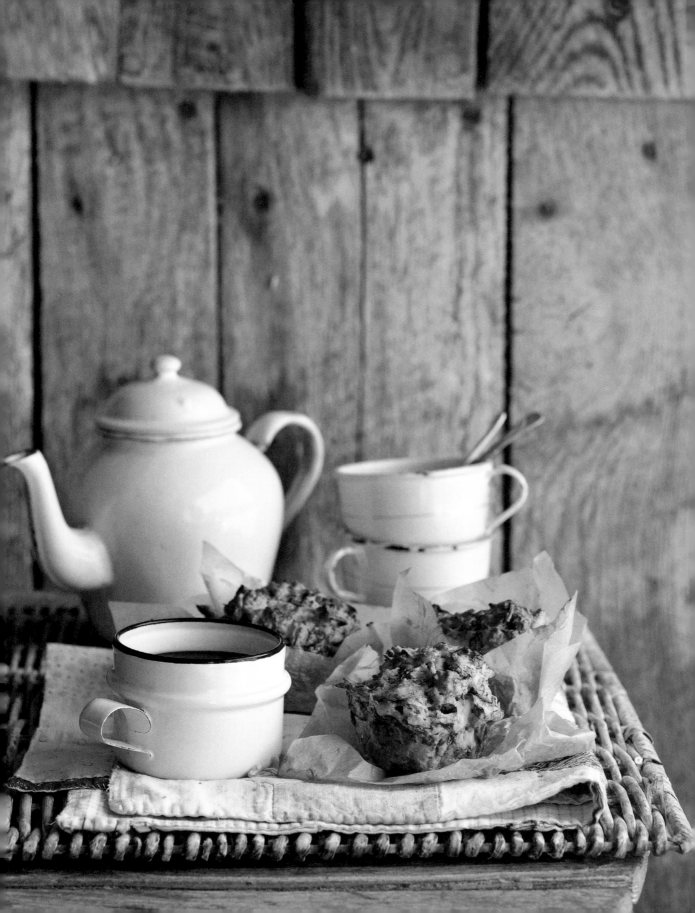

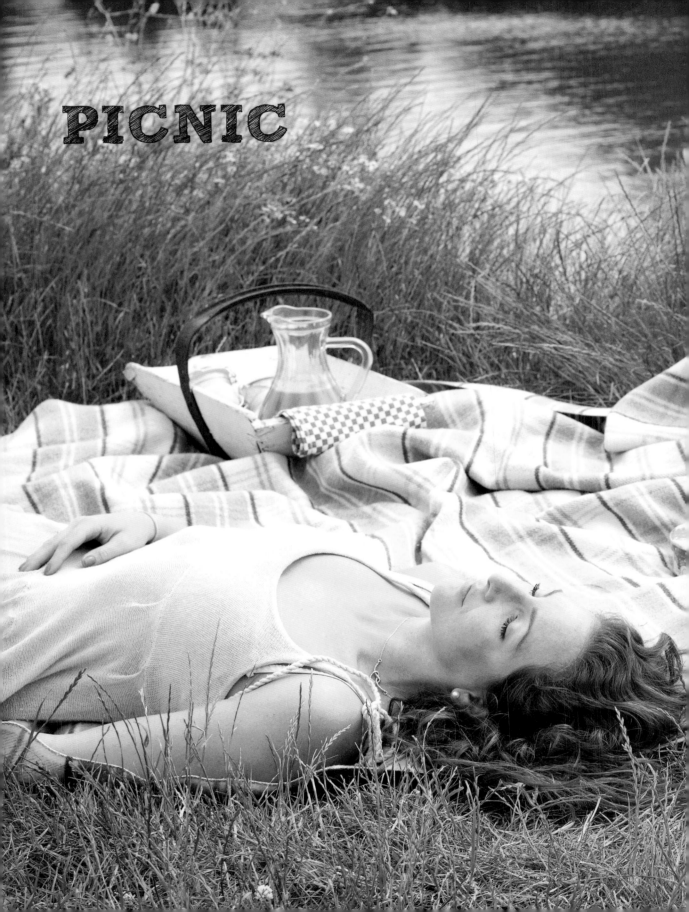

PICNIC

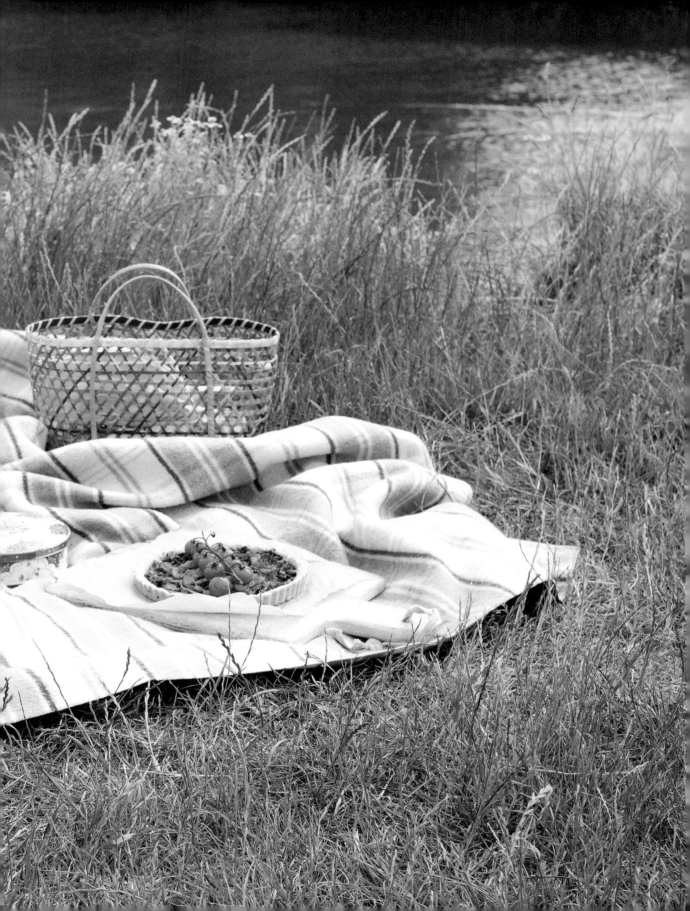

PEA AND MINT SOUP

This soup is perfect for summer—simply transport in a vacuum flask to a picnic destination. This has always been one of my favorite soup recipes and it's so flavorful I could eat it every day!

serves 2

1 tbsp bouillon powder

2½ cups boiling water

1 tbsp sunflower oil

1 white onion, finely chopped

1 bay leaf

3 cups frozen garden peas

½ tsp umeboshi plum purée

½ oz mint, plus extra to garnish

finely grated lemon zest, to garnish

Add the bouillon powder to the boiling water to make a vegetable stock and stir until all the powder has dissolved. Set aside.

Heat the sunflower oil in a pan over medium heat. Sauté the onion and bay leaf until the onions become translucent. Add the frozen peas and stock to the pan then take off the heat after 5 minutes, to ensure you keep the peas' bright green color. Remove the bay leaf, add the umeboshi plum purée and mint, and stir.

Transfer the contents of the pan to a blender. Blend until wonderfully smooth. If you're serving the soup cold, put it in the refrigerator to chill, or warm through if you're serving it hot.

Garnish with lemon zest and fresh mint, and serve.

♥ ♥ Picnic Pleasure

Thirst-quenching juices that provide a hint of natural sweetness are perfect to serve with summer picnics, as they can be made in advance, and stored in vacuum flasks to take to the picnic still slightly chilled. And why not serve a healthy juice that packs in the nutrients at the same time as tasting delicious!

MAKES 4 SMALL OR 2 LARGE GLASSES

4 medium carrots, juiced

2 cucumbers, semi peeled, and juiced (the peel can be quite bitter)

½ pineapple, skin removed, and juiced

1 handful of fresh mint, juiced, plus extra leaves to decorate

Mix all the ingredients together, and add around generous 2 cups of water, if the combination is too strong. Think of the juice as a cordial, and adjust to taste. Serve chilled with sprigs of fresh mint added to each glass.

TASH'S TIPS

This soup is perfect on a summer's day, but works equally well as a warm soup on colder days. Add a swirl of sesame seed paste for an extra protein kick.

NUTRITIONAL NUGGET

Peas contain abundant vitamin C, protein, and vitamin K to support healthy bones and teeth.

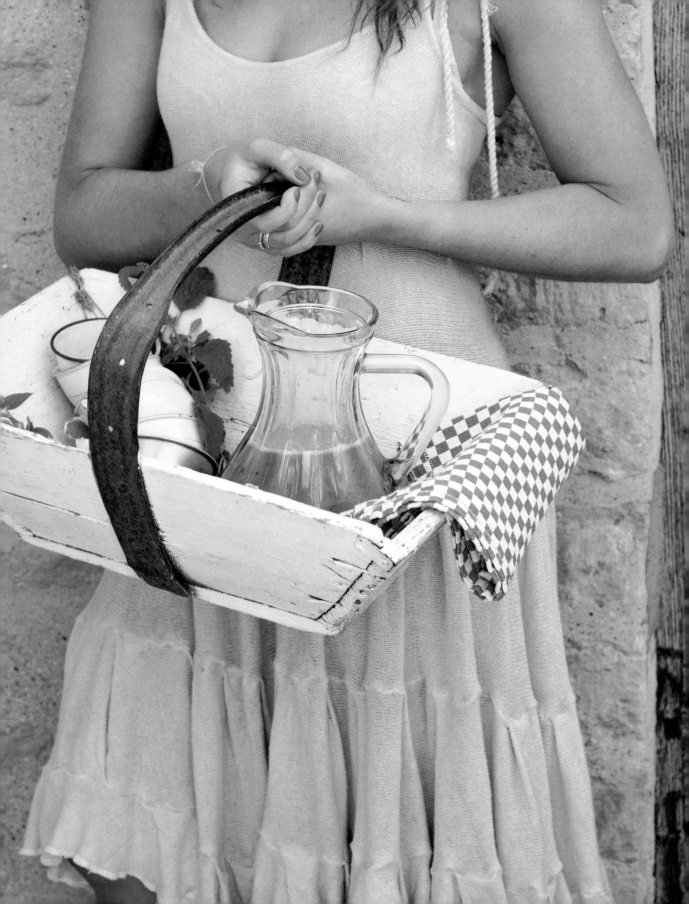

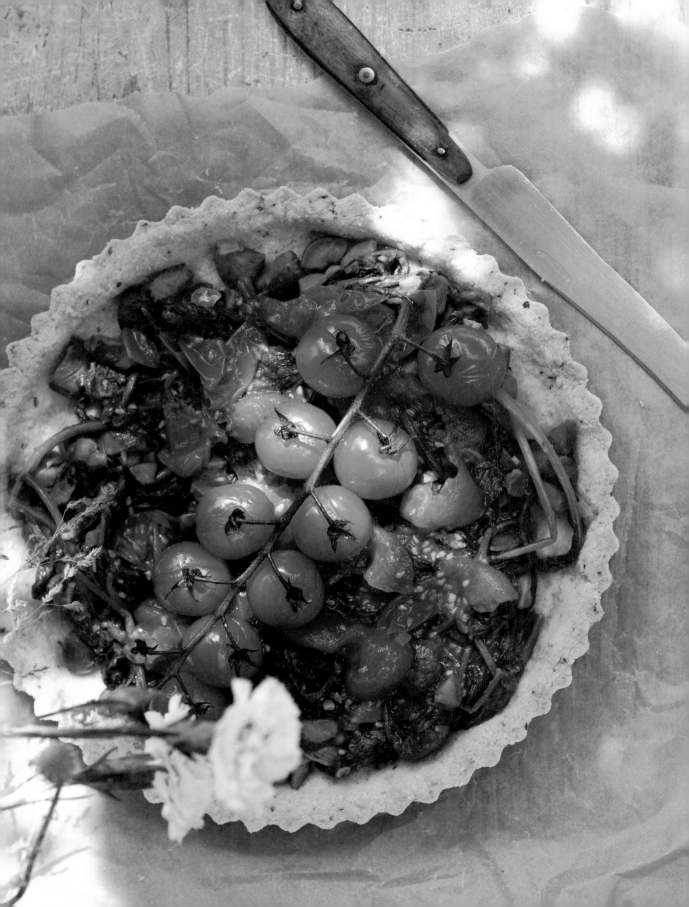

CHESTNUT TART

*I love this tart base as it's so versatile—and I'm sure
you will, too. Once you've tried this chestnut version,
play around with other fillings. Chestnuts work
especially well here as they are so velvety in texture
when cooked. My top tip is to pour the filling into
the base just before you eat it, as otherwise the base
can easily become soggy.*

serves 4

For the crust:

4 tbsp sunflower oil

1 sprig of rosemary, finely chopped

¼ tsp salt

1 tbsp water

2¼ cups ground almonds

For the filling:

7 oz baby vine tomatoes, left on the vine

2 tbsp sunflower oil

1 clove garlic, finely chopped

2 tbsp red onion, finely chopped

4 oz cooked whole chestnuts, finely chopped

½ cup water

⅛ tsp celery seeds

a pinch of Himalayan pink salt

7 oz baby spinach leaves

juice of ½ lemon

1 sprig of basil (optional)

Preheat the oven to 325°F. You'll need a 6-inch tart
pan and a baking sheet.

To make the crust, in a large bowl mix the
sunflower oil, rosemary, salt, and water into the
ground almonds. Press the dough down in the pan
evenly to complete the base and sides. Bake in a
preheated oven for 15 minutes.

Meanwhile, put the tomatoes onto a baking sheet
and drizzle over 1 tablespoon of the sunflower oil
and bake for 10 minutes (while the crust is baking),
until they start to burst and their skins wrinkle.
Once the crust is ready (starts to brown), take it out
of the oven and put into the refrigerator to cool.
Remove the tomatoes from the oven and set aside.

Heat the remaining sunflower oil in a pan on low to
medium heat and sauté the garlic and onions for
2 minutes, then add the chestnuts and half the
measured water. Continue to sauté for another 1 to
2 minutes, until the water is absorbed. Next, add
the celery seeds, a pinch of salt, and the rest of the
measured water. Add the baby spinach and lemon
juice and cook until the leaves are wilted. Once the
spinach leaves are wilted and the liquid is
absorbed, remove the pan from the heat.

Take the tart crust out of the refrigerator and
spoon the mixture into the center.

Take half of the roasted tomatoes off the vine, "pop"
them open in your hands, and carefully place them
onto the tart filling.

Leave the other half of the tomatoes on the vine and
place on top of the tart. Add an extra garnish—a
sprig of basil—if you like.

PEACH AND BUTTERNUT SALAD

This salad screams summertime—it's fresh, refreshing, and zingy all in one. What's more, it's a real crowd pleaser—it's visually stunning and the textures work really well together. However, the secret is that it's so easy. So, here's to making you look like a pro without trying too hard!

serves 3 to 4 as an appetizer or 2 as a main dish

For the salad:
1 butternut squash (you need around 7 oz roasted squash)
1 tsp sunflower oil
3 ripe medium-sized peaches
1 large handful of wild arugula
1¼ oz feta cheese
3 tbsp dill, chopped
finely grated zest of 1 lemon

For the dressing:
3 tbsp dill, chopped
4 tbsp olive oil
1 tbsp rice vinegar
½ tsp brown rice syrup
a pinch of Himalayan pink salt
juice of 1 lemon

Preheat the oven to 350°F.

Peel the squash, cut into quarters, and coat in the sunflower oil. Roast for 30 to 40 minutes. Remove from the oven and set aside.

Slice the peaches and the roasted squash and place on top of a bed of arugula leaves.

Crumble feta cheese and sprinkle the dill and lemon zest over the top.

To make the dressing, simply whisk all the ingredients together and pour over the salad.

TASH'S TIPS
Be sure to pick the ripest of peaches for this recipe. And, if you want, dice up the squash and peaches to create a chopped salad for a change.

NUTRITIONAL NUGGET
Peaches originate from the rose family and are a great source of vitamin C and beta-carotene to support your immune system.

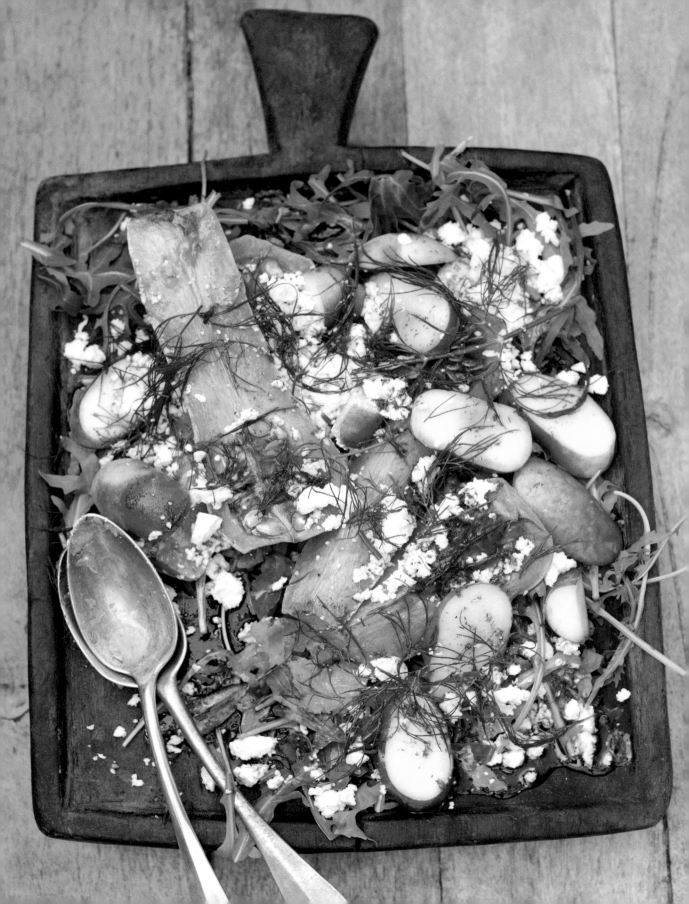

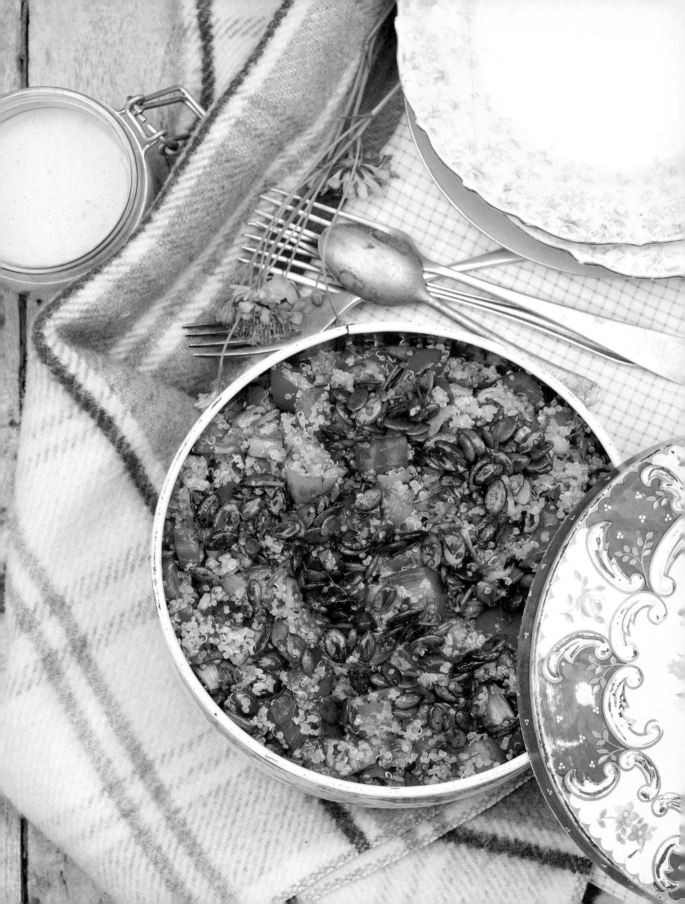

RAINBOW SALAD WITH ROASTED VEGETABLES

Whether served hot or cold, this salad is a riot of color and of taste. You can make all the different components at different times and simply mix together when you are ready to eat. Bear in mind, though, that the pomegranate seeds will dye the quinoa, so only mix them in when you want to eat otherwise the vibrant pink will become dull.

serves 4

1 cup quinoa

2–3 medium-sized carrots, in ½-in cubes

4 tbsp sunflower oil

1 sprig thyme

¾ tsp ground cinnamon

1 red bell pepper, in ½-in cubes

1 yellow bell pepper, in ½-in cubes

Himalayan pink salt, to season

ground black pepper, to season

1 tbsp agave syrup

1 tbsp tamari

scant ½ cup pumpkin seeds

1 clove garlic, finely chopped

1 red onion, finely chopped

1 leek, finely chopped

¾ cup chervil, chopped

¾ cup cilantro, chopped

finely grated zest of 1 lemon

1 pomegranate

For the dressing:

3 tbsp sweet miso

2 tbsp sesame seed paste

1 tbsp sesame oil

4 tbsp water

Preheat the oven to 350°F. You'll need three baking sheets.

Cook the quinoa according to the package instructions but overcook slightly, so it's fluffy; this should take around 20 minutes. Drain off the remaining water and set aside.

In one baking sheet, toss the carrots in 1 tablespoon of oil, along with the fresh thyme and ½ teaspoon of cinnamon. Roast in the preheated oven for 25 minutes.

In a separate baking sheet, toss the pepper pieces with 1 tablespoon of oil along with some pink salt and black pepper. After 15 minutes of the carrots being in the oven, put the peppers in for the final 10 minutes.

Next, mix together the agave syrup, sunflower oil, and tamari, coat the pumpkin seeds, and toast in the third sheet for the final 5 minutes in the oven.

Meanwhile, heat the remaining oil in a skillet on low heat and add the garlic and onions. As the oil starts to be absorbed, add a splash of water (around 1 tablespoon) to cool the pan, then add the leeks. Sauté for 2 minutes, until the onions become translucent and soft. Remove from the heat.

Take all the baking sheets out of the oven; they should have all completed their cooking time by now. Mix all the vegetables (both the ones on the baking sheets and the skillet, but not the toasted seeds) with the fresh herbs and add ¼ teaspoon of cinnamon and the lemon zest. Stir this into the quinoa and set aside.

Bang the seeds out of the pomegranate and set aside. (There will be a little juice left in the bottom, don't throw it away—drink it, it's so good for you!) Add half the pomegranate seeds to the salad and mix in. Serve garnished with the toasted pumpkin seeds and the remaining pomegranate seeds.

Finally, whisk all the dressing ingredients together and then drizzle over the top.

PUY LENTIL AND POMEGRANATE SALSA RAW "NOODLES"

It's good to know you can whip up this beautiful and delicious dish in no time at all. If you haven't got time to cook your own Puy lentils you can use canned ones to make life easier for you. I find these are great for picnics and for lunch on-the-go, too.

serves 2

1 zucchini

1 cup cooked Puy lentils

seeds of ½ pomegranate

1 tsp chervil, chopped finely

1 tsp dill, chopped finely

5–7 drops each of mirin, brown rice vinegar, and toasted sesame oil

sunflower seeds, to garnish

For the dressing:

1 tbsp sesame seed paste

2 tbsp water

¼ tsp umeboshi plum purée

juice of ½ lime

Using a spiralizer, spiralize your zucchini (see also page 74) and put on a serving plate.

In a bowl, put the cooked lentils, pomegranate seeds, fresh chopped herbs, mirin, brown rice vinegar, and toasted sesame oil and mix together.

In a cup, make the dressing. Whisk the sesame seed paste with the water until smooth—don't worry if it looks like it's curdling, just whisk faster. Next, add the umeboshi plum purée and lime juice and mix again.

Pour the dressing over the lentils and mix well. Serve over the raw zucchini "noodles" and sprinkle with sunflower seeds.

TASH'S TIPS

A spiralizer is a fantastic kitchen implement but also a great toy—so this is one to get the kids involved in. If you like, you can also spiralize carrots, which adds an extra color and texture to the dish.

NUTRITIONAL NUGGET

Pomegranates have abundant insoluble fiber and contain most of the B-complex vitamins, vital for energy. The seeds and juice provide antioxidants, vitamin C, and ellagic acid, for great heart health.

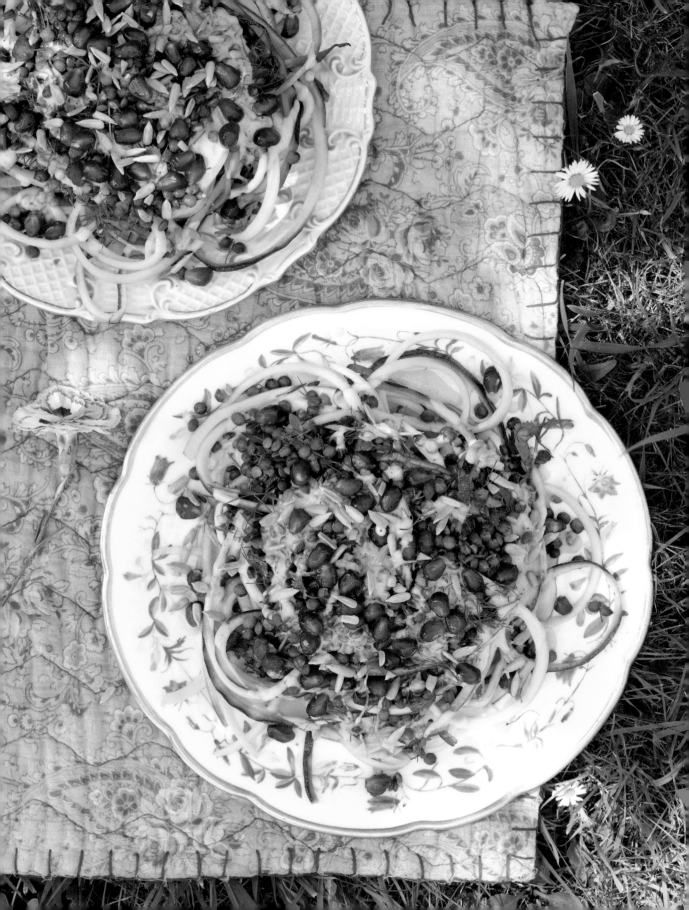

TEA PARTY

ORANGE AND ANISEED TEACAKES

These ultra-light mouthfuls are perfect for afternoon tea and are something different to impress your guests with. If you don't have molds for tea cakes you could always use a mini loaf pan or silicone cupcake holders instead.

serves 2

For the teacakes:
5 tbsp aniseeds
⅓ cup orange juice
2 eggs
1⅔ cups ground almonds
scant ⅓ cup goat's yogurt
2½ tbsp date syrup
¼ tsp vanilla extract
½ tsp baking soda
finely grated zest of 1 orange

For the drizzle:
1 tbsp aniseeds
juice of 2 oranges
2 tbsp date syrup

Preheat the oven to 350°F, and grease two 4-inch Savarin or baby Bundt tins.

Whiz up 3 tablespoons of the aniseeds in a coffee grinder until a coarse powder. Lightly toast the remaining whole aniseeds in a skillet. When they start to brown, add the orange juice and continue to heat until the liquid has reduced right down—this should only take a minute. Set aside.

In a bowl, whisk the eggs and then add the ground almonds, ground aniseed, goat's yogurt, date syrup, vanilla extract, and baking soda and mix to combine. Then stir through the whole aniseed and any remaining orange juice. Add the orange zest and mix through.

Spoon the batter into the greased tins and bake in a preheated oven for 20 minutes.

Remove the cakes from the oven and transfer to a wire rack to cool.

To make the drizzle, put all the ingredients into a pan and bring to a simmer for 3 to 5 minutes, until the sauce thickens. Then pour over the tea cakes and enjoy with a lovely cup of mint tea.

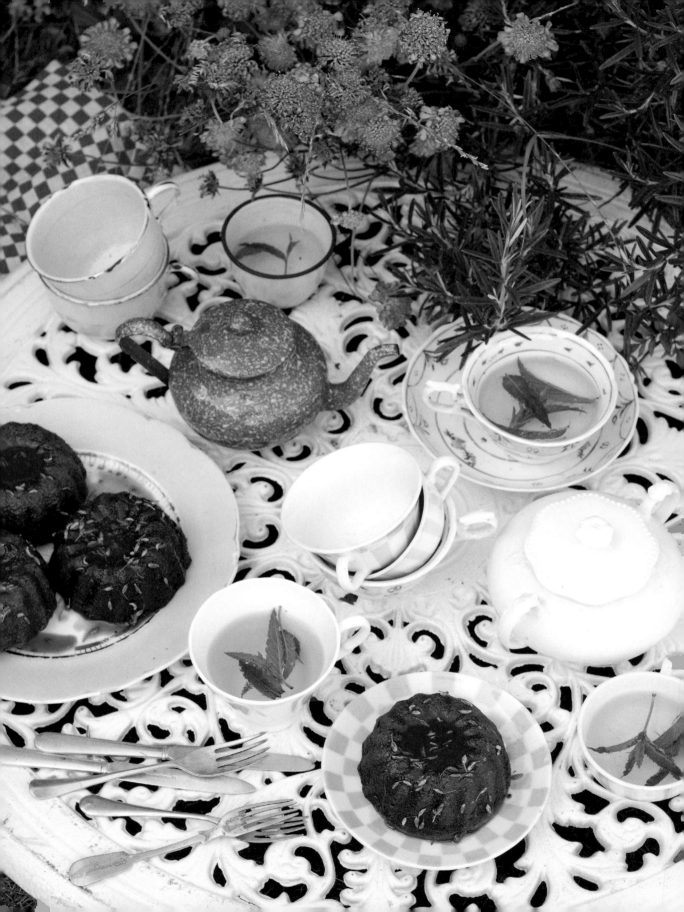

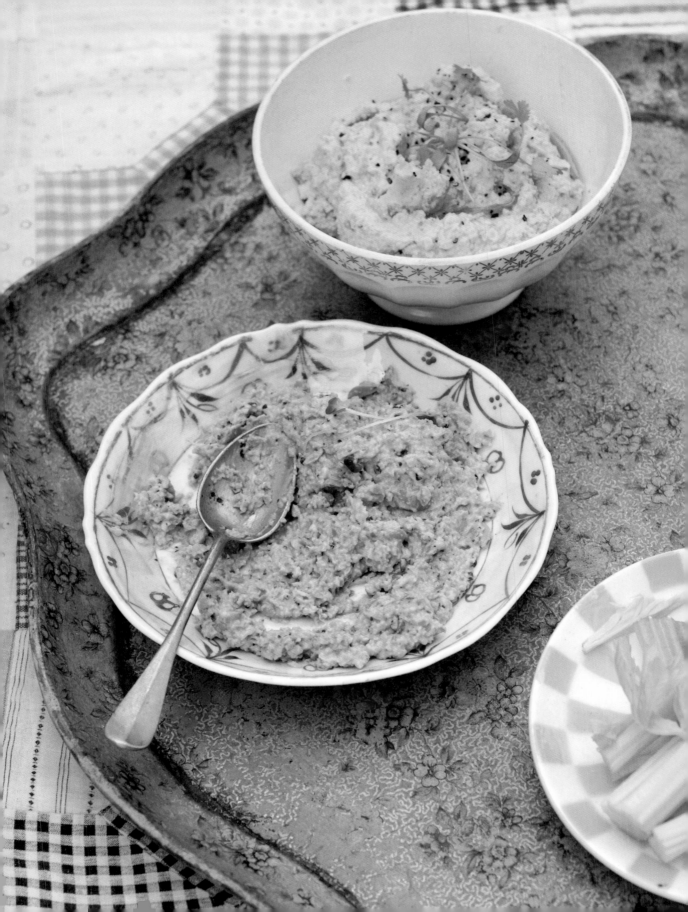

EASY EDAMAME DIP

As well as being easy to prepare, this vibrant soy bean dip works well for a perfectly healthy afternoon snack, a dinner party hors d'oeuvres, or a quick-fix for Sunday night.

serves 8 to 10
1 lb 2 oz frozen edamame (podded), defrosted
finely grated zest and juice of 1 lemon
½ tsp Himalayan pink salt
4 tbsp sesame seed paste
1 clove garlic
scant ½ cup olive oil
½ oz mint

In a blender or food processor, pulse two-thirds of the edamame with the lemon zest, juice, salt, sesame seed paste, garlic, and olive oil till smooth.

Add in the remaining edamame along with the mint and pulse for a couple of seconds to give the dip a lovely chunky texture. And it's done.

MY FAMOUS HUMMUS

Everyone always asks me for my recipe for hummus, so here it is... This spiced chickpea dip is a perfect protein snack. (If you don't have time to soak dried chickpeas, you can always use half the quantity of canned chickpeas.) I like to make a batch up on a Sunday night to get ready for the week, but you could easily whiz some together for a Saturday picnic and use the rest for weekday lunches or a nibble when you get in from work. Once you're happy with how to make it and its taste, why not try it with different flavors—mix some puréed spinach or fresh herbs into it.

serves 8 to 10
2¼ cups dried chickpeas
1 piece kombu seaweed
1 heaping tsp ground cumin
1 clove garlic
scant ½ cup olive oil
scant ½ cup water
scant ½ cup sesame seed paste
scant ¼ cup lemon juice

Soak the chickpeas overnight (around 12 hours), drain them, and then boil them with fresh water and the kombu seaweed until they are al dente.

Drain them and discard the piece of kombu. While the chickpeas are still warm, put them into a food processor along with all the other ingredients.

Pulse until smooth and enjoy with raw vegetable crudités or wheat-free crackers.

NUTRITIONAL NUGGET

Beans can be hard to digest as our bodies don't have the right enzyme to do this. Kombu seaweed, however, contains exactly the right enzyme to break down the oligosaccharides (complex sugars) in the beans, thereby making them much more digestible and less likely to cause bloating and gas.

VELVETY BOUNTY BARS

*This recipe was one of those that I stumbled on by
chance. When I bit into one of these for the first time,
childhood memories of eating Bounty bars—similar
to Mounds candy bars for you Americans—came
flooding back. So, now you don't have to miss out on
that luxurious coconutty chocolate dream, you can
make a batch and reach for this healthy version.*

makes 24

For the filling:
½ cup raw cashew nuts
8 tbsp dry unsweetened coconut
1 tbsp coconut oil
3 tbsp xylitol

For the chocolate:
1 cup raw cacao butter
¾ cup raw cacao powder
⅓ cup agave syrup
½ tsp vanilla extract

Soak the cashews for 1 hour in water that just
covers them and then drain.

In a blender or food processor, whiz all the
ingredients for the filling together to give a
textured paste. Push teaspoonfuls of the mixture
into a silicone ice-cube tray and put into the freezer
for 1 hour.

Meanwhile, melt the raw cacao butter in a
heatproof bowl over a pan of simmering water, or
in a bain marie, and then let cool for around
10 minutes. Next, mix in the cacao powder. Once
incorporated, add the agave and vanilla extract.

Leave the chocolate to cool down, until it's thick
enough to run off the back of a spoon—this thicker
chocolate will give your bars a wonderful coating.

Take the filling mixture out of the freezer and pop
the shapes out of the ice-cube tray. Dip them into
the chocolate mixture, one at a time, taking them
out with a fork so that they are covered all over.
Put them onto a baking sheet lined with parchment
paper and pop back into the freezer to set for
15 minutes.

These are triple-dipped delights, so take them out
of the freezer, dip in the chocolate, and return to
the freezer to set twice more, and then keep them
in the freezer until you're ready to eat them.

The chocolate coating for these Bounty bars also
makes the perfect dipping chocolate for fruit of all
kinds, as you'll see on the endpapers of this book
(that's right inside the back cover).

TASH'S TIPS
Hide these in the freezer, out of sight,
as they are so delicious you will want
to eat them all!

NUTRITIONAL NUGGET
Dry unsweetened coconut is rich in
protein and cholesterol-lowering
essential fats.

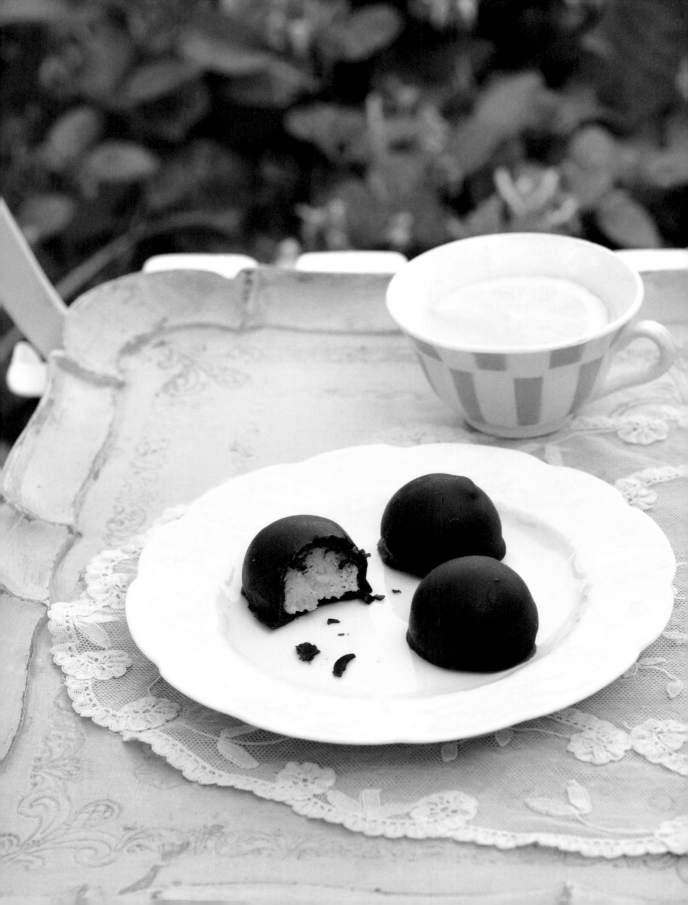

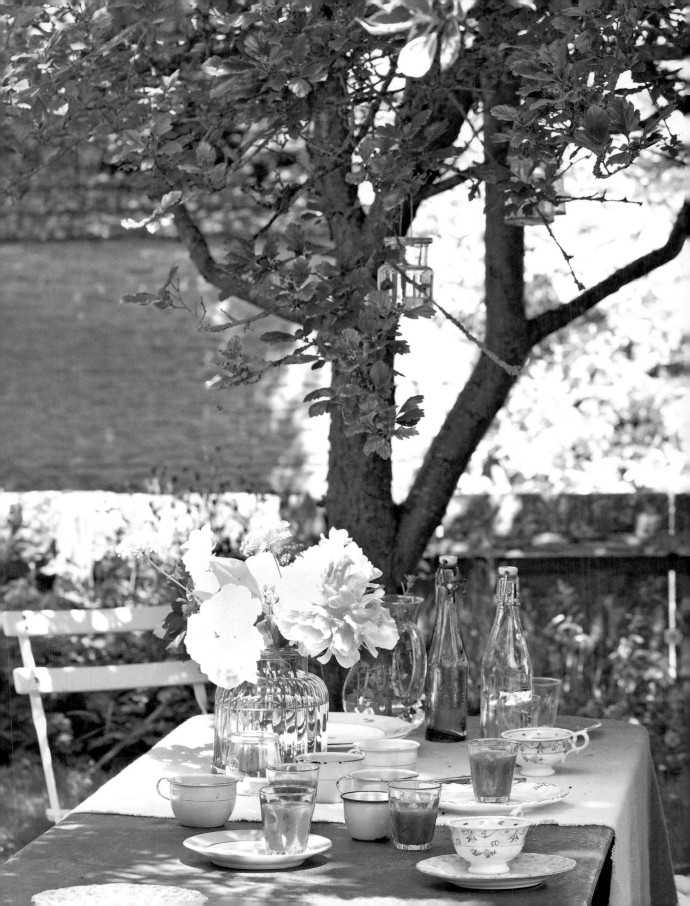

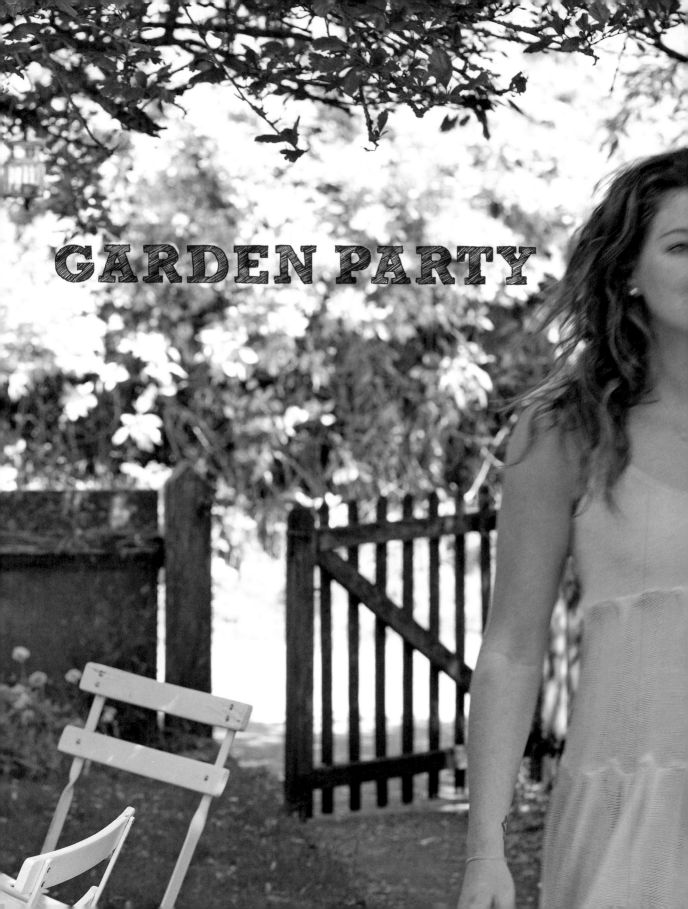

GARDEN PARTY

WATERMELON GAZPACHO

I love gazpacho, but sometimes it's good to tweak the old classics. This recipe came about when I was on vacation in Spain, someone offered me a gazpacho and I already had a plate of watermelon sitting in front of me...well, my brain started working overtime and watermelon gazpacho was the result! You could serve this with some delicious herbed ice cubes to keep it nice and cool .

serves 4 to 6

15 oz watermelon

1 large vine tomato (around 7 oz)

1 red bell pepper

3½ oz cucumber, peeled

⅛ tsp fresh chili

¼ tsp grated fresh ginger

1 celery stalk

juice of 2 limes

¾ oz cilantro

Put all the ingredients apart from the cilantro into a blender and blend until smooth. Then add the cilantro and pulse just for a few seconds.

Serve super-chilled either in shot glasses for a canapé or in bowls for a delicious appetizer.

NUTRITIONAL NUGGET

Watermelon is drenched in vitamin C as well as potassium, making it one of the most alkaline fruits.

DECORATIVE ICE CUBES

These add such a lovely touch to any table arrangement—especially for a gathering in the garden—and also add scrumptious flavors when they start to melt. All you need is an ice-cube tray and a selection of herbs, edible flowers, or fruit. My favorite combo is mint, lemon, and rose petals.

Suggested ingredients

Leafy herbs

   such as mint, thyme, basil, and rosemary

Citrus fruits

   such as lemons and oranges as thin strips of zest

Edible flowers

   such as violets, nasturtiums, and jasmine

Berries

   such as blueberries and redcurrants

Flower petals

   such as roses, daisies, and buttercups

Rose water

   a few drops for a hint of taste

Orange-flower water

   a few drops for a hint of taste

Chop up any herbs coarsely and place them into an ice-cube tray. Carefully pour in the water and pop in the freezer until set. I often make mine a few days ahead.

For those ingredients you want to keep whole—berries, flowers, and flower petals—just arrange in the ice-cube tray or source other molds that might suit them better. As above, carefully pour in the water and pop in the freezer until set.

To add a hint of flavor, add a few drops of rose water or orange-flower water.

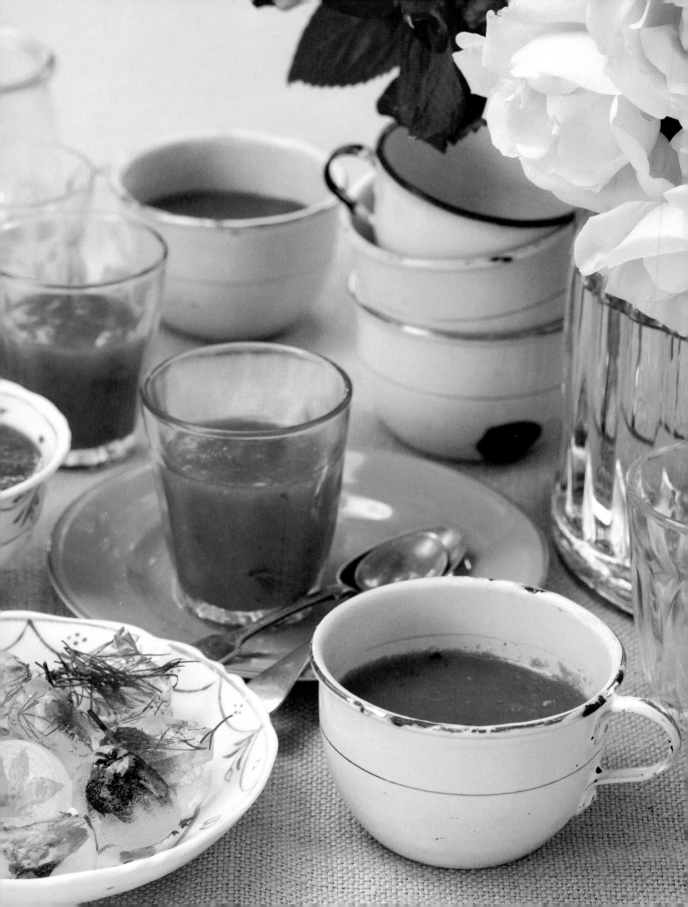

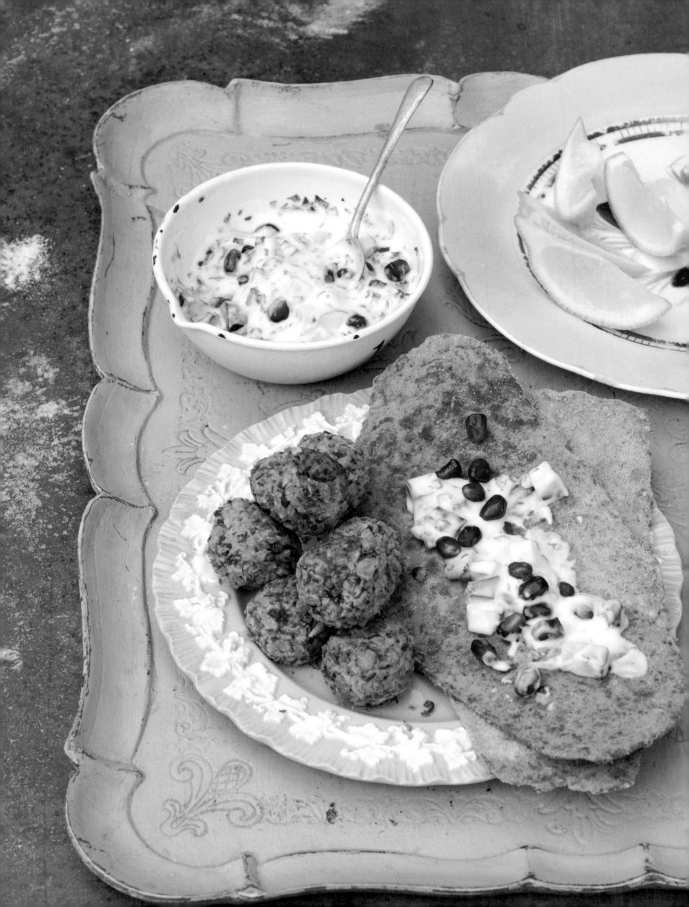

LENTIL FALAFEL WITH BUCKWHEAT FLATBREADS

My idea here was to create a new and different-tasting falafel. And I hope you agree this fits the bill. It's a great healthy alternative to fried falafel and utterly delicious with the flatbread. You can use the flatbread with all the dips in this book, or even as an open sandwich for a nice change.

serves 8 to 10

½ leek

½ red onion

1 clove garlic

1 tsp sesame oil

1 cup cooked Puy lentils

½ cup cooked chickpeas

⅓ cup raw sunflower seeds

5 tbsp hummus (see page 211)

Himalayan pink salt, to taste

pomegranate seeds, to garnish (optional)

Preheat the oven to 325°F and line a baking sheet with parchment paper.

Slice the leek and red onion as finely as you can, or use a mandolin, and crush the garlic. In a skillet over medium heat add the oil and sauté the vegetables until soft. Take the skillet off the heat and set aside to cool.

Put the lentils, chickpeas, and sunflower seeds into a food processor and pulse for 1 minute.

Add the blitzed legumes and seeds to the softened vegetables and add the hummus to bind the mixture together, adding salt to taste.

Form the mixture into balls around 2 inches in diameter and place on the prepared baking sheet.

Bake in the preheated oven for 15 minutes. Remove from the oven and transfer to a serving plate and serve while hot, with the flatbreads on the side, some Herby Yogurt Dressing (see page 82) and a smattering of pomegranate seeds.

Buckwheat flatbreads

makes 16 flatbreads

1 cup buckwheat flour, plus extra for rolling out

1 cup ground chia seeds

1 tsp Himalayan pink salt

2 tsp mixed herbs

5 tsp baking powder

5 tsp caraway seeds

8 eggs

sunflower oil, for frying

Mix all the dry ingredients together in a bowl and make a well in the center. Crack all the eggs into the well and then, using one hand to hold the bowl and one hand to stir, mix all the ingredients together to form a ball of dough.

Allow the dough to rest at room temperature for 15 minutes. Then, divide the ball of dough into 16 smaller balls.

Dust your counter or a wooden board and a rolling pin with some buckwheat flour. Place one small ball of dough onto the floured surface, sprinkle more buckwheat flour over the ball, and roll it out into a thin flatbread shape. Repeat with the remaining balls of dough.

Put a large skillet over high heat. Dab some paper towel in a little sunflower oil and quickly wipe around the hot pan.

Place two flatbreads in the pan and cook them for 1½ to 2 minutes then flip over and cook the other side. If you like, set aside on a warm plate while you cook the rest of the flatbreads, but they are equally delicious cold. Be sure to wipe the pan with the oily paper towel before cooking each new pair of flatbreads.

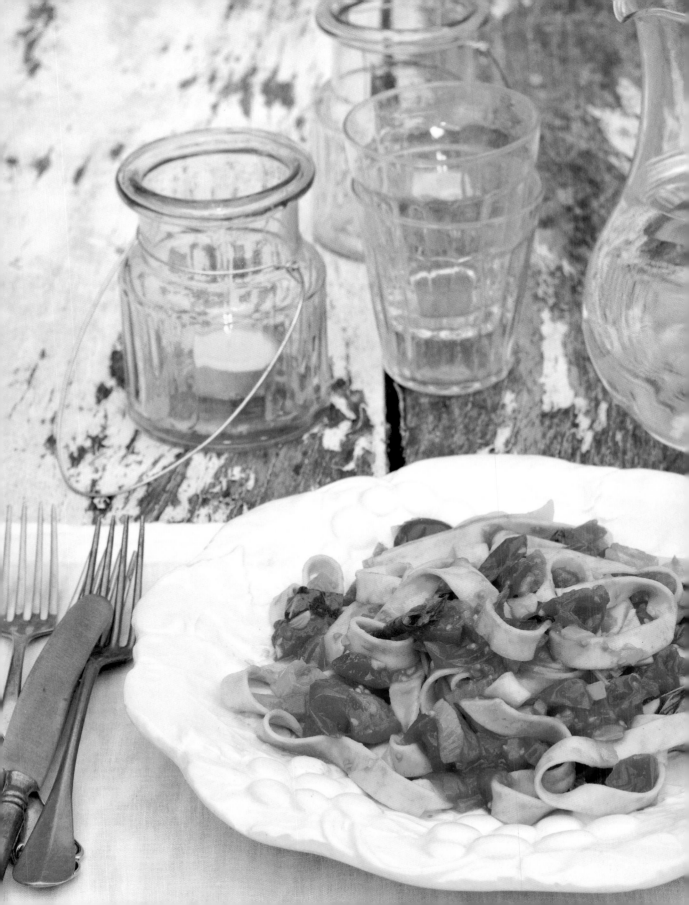

A GREAT TOMATO SAUCE FOR PASTA

This tomato sauce was a staple in our household and my stepfather Huggy taught me how to make it... this may not be quite as spicy as his version, but it is equally delicious!

serves 2

2 tbsp sunflower oil

1 clove garlic, crushed

½ onion, chopped into small cubes

2½ cup water

12½ oz vine tomatoes, chopped in half

¼ tsp balsamic vinegar

½ tsp umeboshi plum purée

½-in fresh red chili (optional)

1 oz basil

2 tbsp coconut milk

Heat the sunflower oil in a pan over medium heat. Add the garlic and onion and cook for 2 minutes.

Measure out ½ cup of the water and add to the onions and garlic. Let the onions absorb the water then add 1 cup of water. Next, add the vine tomatoes, balsamic vinegar, umeboshi plum purée, and the rest of the measured water. Simmer over medium to low heat for 10 minutes.

Add the fresh chili, if you like a spicy kick, and stir in half of the basil and the coconut milk. The sauce should be reducing nicely now.

Leave to simmer for another 5 to 7 minutes. If you like a runny sauce add a little extra water, if needed; reduce it further if you prefer a drier and more intense sauce.

Cook the pasta (I use gluten-free or spelt pasta) according to the package instructions. Once cooked, mix with the sauce along with the remaining basil leaves and serve straightaway.

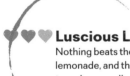

Luscious Lemonade

Nothing beats the refreshing taste of homemade lemonade, and this recipe is ridiculously simple to make, as well as being wholly alkaline.

MAKES 4 SMALL OR 2 LARGE GLASSES

4 cups alkaline or filtered water

juice of 2 lemons, strained

a thumb-sized piece of ginger root, peeled, grated, and squeezed

a small pinch of Himalayan pink salt

2 tsp raw honey or agave nectar

Mix all the ingredients thoroughly, and chill slightly before serving with herb or flower ice cubes (see page 216).

Optional alcoholic version: Double the amount of lemon juice and salt, and serve over crushed ice, adding 1 shot of vodka per person. Portion guide: 1 shot of vodka to 3 shots of lemonade.

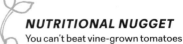

NUTRITIONAL NUGGET

You can't beat vine-grown tomatoes for beta-carotene—one of the most powerful antioxidants that protect skin from aging prematurely.

HUGGY'S ICE CREAM

The reason I call my stepfather, Ed, Huggy is because when I was little he used to always eat Häagen–Dazs ice cream and could eat a whole tub in one sitting! But he is also incredibly huggable! So, this ice cream is for my Huggy, a recipe he loves to make himself that I have adapted slightly. Be sure to make your ice cream at least a day ahead of when you want to eat it. Serve in a bowl or in a sugar-free and gluten-free ice cream cone.

makes 6⅓ cups

4 cups coconut milk

⅓ cup agave syrup

3 oz dates, pitted

1 tbsp raw cacao powder

3 tbsp water

⅓ cup raw cacao nibs

Put the ice-cream bowl of an ice-cream machine into the freezer the day before you want to make your ice cream.

In a pan over medium heat, bring the coconut milk to a boil, add in the agave syrup, stir, and then take it off the heat. Put this mixture into the refrigerator to cool down; transfer to a bowl or just put the pan in the refrigerator, it's up to you.

Meanwhile, put the dates, raw cacao powder, and the water into a high-speed blender, or food processer, and blitz until everything roughly comes together.

Once your bowl is frozen and your coconut milk mixture is cold, you can start making your ice cream. Pour the coconut milk mixture into the ice-cream machine's bowl and pour in the raw cacao nibs as well, switch it on, and let it churn for 10 minutes. Then add the chocolatey date mixture, and let it churn for another 15 minutes. Empty the contents of the ice-cream machine's bowl into an airtight container and freeze for a couple of hours before serving.

TASH'S TIPS
If you don't have an ice-cream maker, be sure to stir the mixture in the freezer frequently to avoid getting icy particles in your gorgeous ice cream.

NUTRITIONAL NUGGET
Cacao nibs are a rich source of iron, protein, and magnesium, as well as tryptophan—the precursor for the neurotransmitter, serotonin, known for its "feel-good" factor.

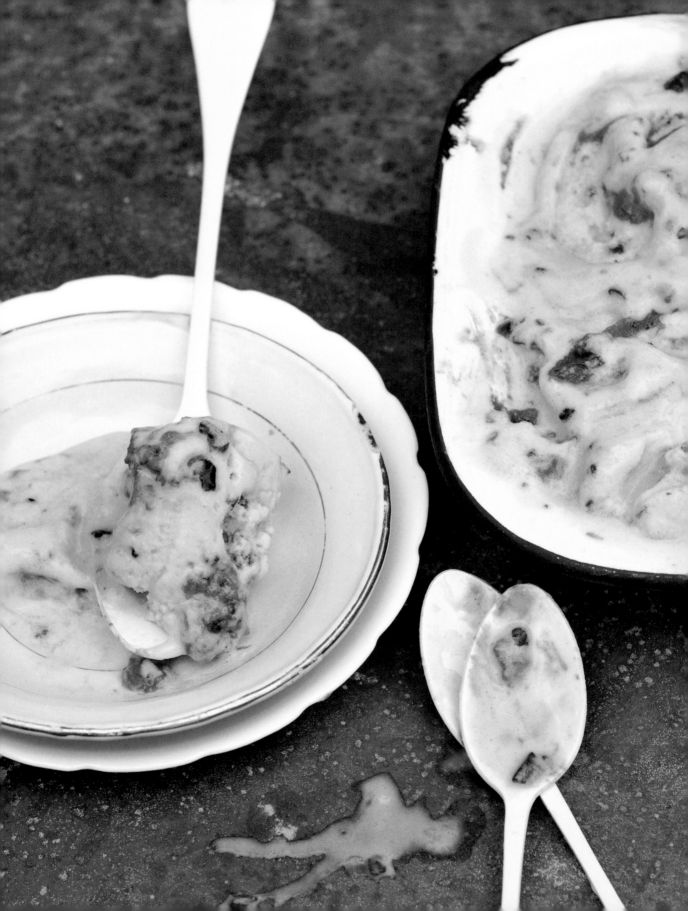

HOSTESS WITH

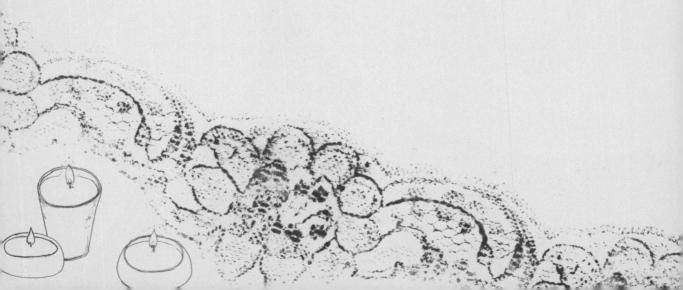

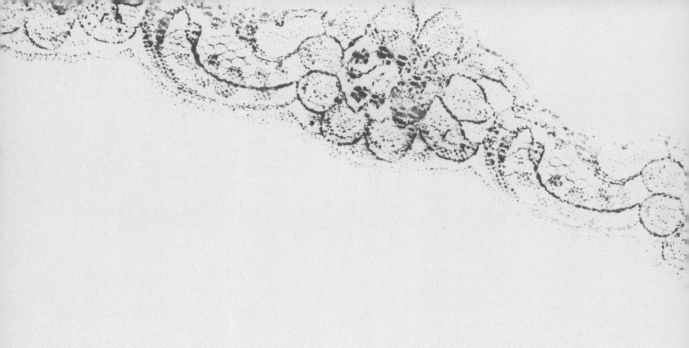

THE MOSTEST

I never consider entertaining a chore, and with this host of recipes under your belt, neither will you. There are plenty of dishes for you to scale up or down as you choose, depending on who's coming for dinner, as well as sigh-inducing nibbles. And just by being organized and doing some work in advance, you'll get to enjoy being the hostess with the mostest.

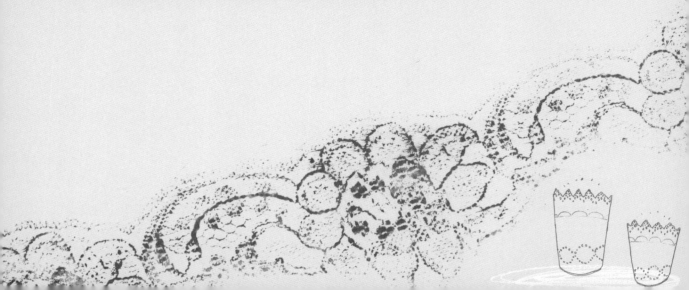

GIRLS' NIGHT IN

SMOKED TOFU AND TAMARIND TOMATO SAUCE WITH BROWN RICE

This dish was inspired by a trip to Vietnam where they love to use tamarind in their food and I love it, too—it's a perfect balance of sweet and sour. Great for a Sunday night sofa dinner with friends or family, and you can eat any leftovers for lunch.

serves 2

scant ½ cup brown rice

2 tbsp sunflower oil

1 clove garlic, chopped

1 small red onion, chopped

¾ cup water

2 oz dried tamarind, soaked, pips removed, and drained

10¼ oz baby vine tomatoes, taken off the vine

¼ tsp balsamic vinegar

5½ oz smoked tofu, in ¾-in cubes

1 scallion, sliced on the diagonal

3 tbsp cilantro, chopped

Cook the brown rice following the package instructions. Meanwhile, heat the sunflower oil in a pan over medium heat. Add the garlic and onion and sauté for 1 to 2 minutes.

Add scant ¼ cup of the measured water along with the tamarind. Cook for 3 minutes then add the remaining water, the whole baby vine tomatoes, and the balsamic vinegar.

Leave to cook over medium heat for another 3 minutes, then add the smoked tofu and the scallion. Cook for another 2 minutes and then take off the heat—the sauce should be thick and all the tomatoes will have burst. (Depending on how long the rice takes to cook, you might want to reheat the sauce just before serving.)

Lastly, stir in the cilantro and serve over brown rice. Garnish with cilantro leaves if you wish.

NUTRITIONAL NUGGET
Tamarind is a great source of natural soluble fiber, as well as providing a nutty sour-sweetness. Being soaked and removed from the original roots preserves their natural nutrients.

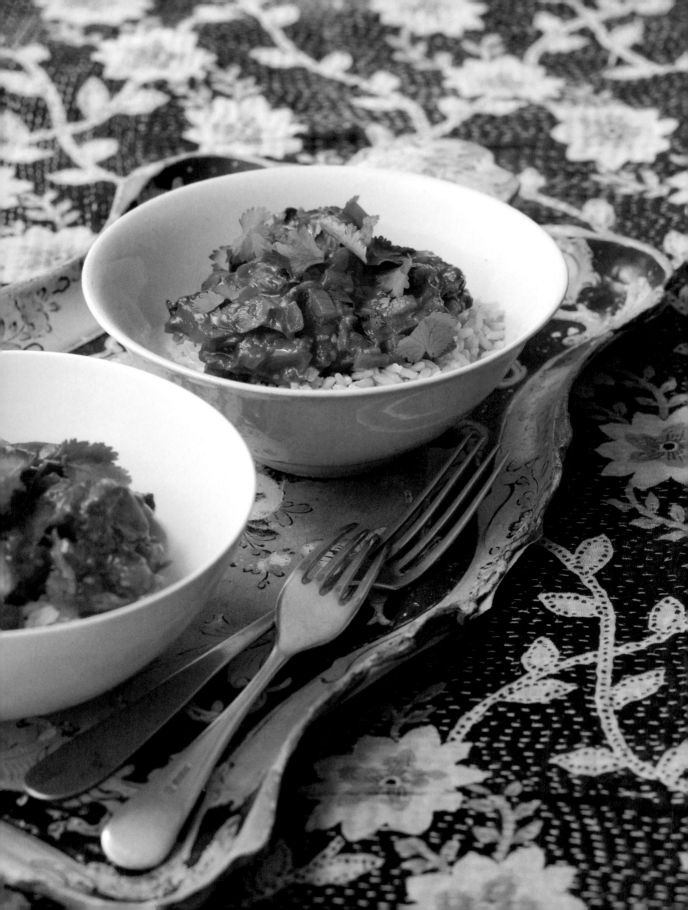

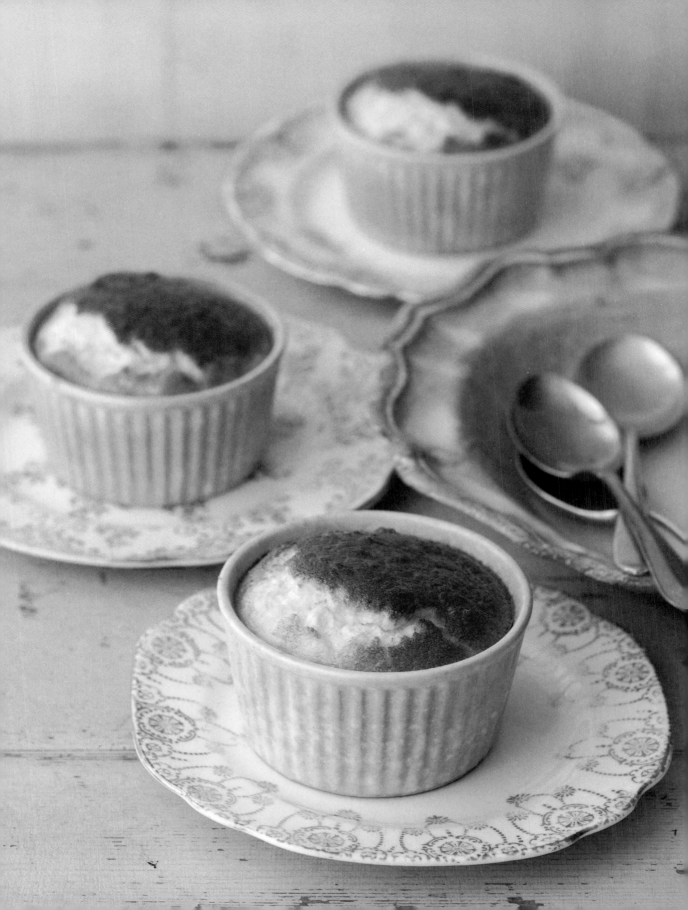

GRANNY'S CHEESE SOUFFLÉS

My wonderful grandmother Stephanie loves all soufflés. She always used to make us her flourless cheese soufflé, so I asked her how to make it and then adapted it to using sheep's and goat's cheese rather than cow's and it worked perfectly. It's so tasty and gives her recipe a run for its money I think!

serves 6

3 oz hard goat's cheese, such as Cheddar

3 oz hard sheep's cheese, such as Pecorino

¾ cup goat's yogurt

½ tsp Dijon mustard

3 egg yolks

6 egg whites

Preheat the oven to 400°F, and set aside six ramekins.

Grate both the cheeses into a large bowl and add the yogurt and mustard and mix well.

Gently whisk the egg yolks with a fork and add them to the bowl with the cheese and yogurt and mix in. Boil some water for a bain marie.

In a separate bowl, whisk the egg whites until stiff peaks form and then gradually add the egg whites into the cheese mixture and gently fold with a silver spoon until incorporated. Spoon the mixture into the ramekins and place them in an empty roasting tin. Pour boiling water from the kettle half way up the ramekins to create the bain marie.

Bake in the preheated oven for 20 to 23 minutes, until beautifully risen and golden brown on top. Remove from the oven and serve immediately.

♥ ♥ Tummy Tonic

Many people need to change the way they eat to alleviate indigestion, and improve their absorption of nutrients from their foods. There is no quicker way of providing a solution than adding raw apple cider vinegar to a juice or drink to stimulate those stomach juices—your friends will thank you for this as they will enjoy their meal all the more! For optimal health, drink a little of this before every meal—and witness the difference in your energy levels straightaway.

MAKES 4 SMALL OR 2 LARGE GLASSES

4 tbsp raw apple cider vinegar (1 tbsp per glass)

6⅓ cups sparkling water

juice of 2 lemons

juice of 2 apples

Combine all the ingredients in a pitcher, and serve as a non-alcoholic mocktail prior to eating—do not add ice, as this drink is best served at room temperature for optimal effect.

TASH'S TIPS

Serve these straightaway as they will deflate when they come out of the oven. And do be really careful when taking them out of the oven as the tin of water is incredibly hot.

NUTRITIONAL NUGGET

Eggs are still considered the ultimate all-rounder, as they contain literally all the nutrients one needs for mind and body. As a source of protein, they are perfect, and no longer carry the cholesterol-stimulating dogma. For vegetarians in particular, they are a super source of all amino acids.

THAI MANGO AND CORN SALAD WITH POMEGRANATE RELISH

I love this salad: it's a perfect appetizer for a dinner party or a casual supper. It's nice and light but it's also really quick to make, so you are not slaving away in the kitchen while your guests enjoy themselves in a room nearby.

serves 2

For the salad:
½ a corn on the cob
1½ oz green mango
1½ oz ripe mango
½ oz scallions
¾ cup bean sprouts
3 tbsp cilantro, roughly chopped
1 small red chili, deseeded and finely sliced
a small handful of mizuna leaves
1 tbsp toasted sesame oil, for searing

For the dressing:
1 small garlic clove, grated
1 small knob of root ginger, grated
juice of ½ lime
a pinch of Himalayan pink salt

For the relish:
3 tbsp cilantro, finely chopped
½ cup pomegranate seeds
a pinch of Himalayan pink salt
¼ tsp lime juice
¼ tsp pomegranate molasses

Put the corn in a pan of boiling water and boil for 10 minutes. Meanwhile, julienne the mangoes and scallion and mix together in a bowl with the bean sprouts, cilantro, chili, and mizuna leaves.

Combine the dressing ingredients together in a separate bowl and then mix through the salad.

When the corn is cooked, remove from the pan and set aside. Heat the toasted sesame oil in a skillet and sear each side of the cob until colored. Chop the cob into four slices, roughly ½-inch thick.

Next, mix together all the relish ingredients.

To serve, pile a handful of salad onto a plate. Top with two slices of corn and a spoonful of relish.

NUTRITIONAL NUGGET
One of the richest sources of beta-carotene and vitamin C, mangoes have an abundance of soluble fiber, and can be eaten in their green or ripe varieties.

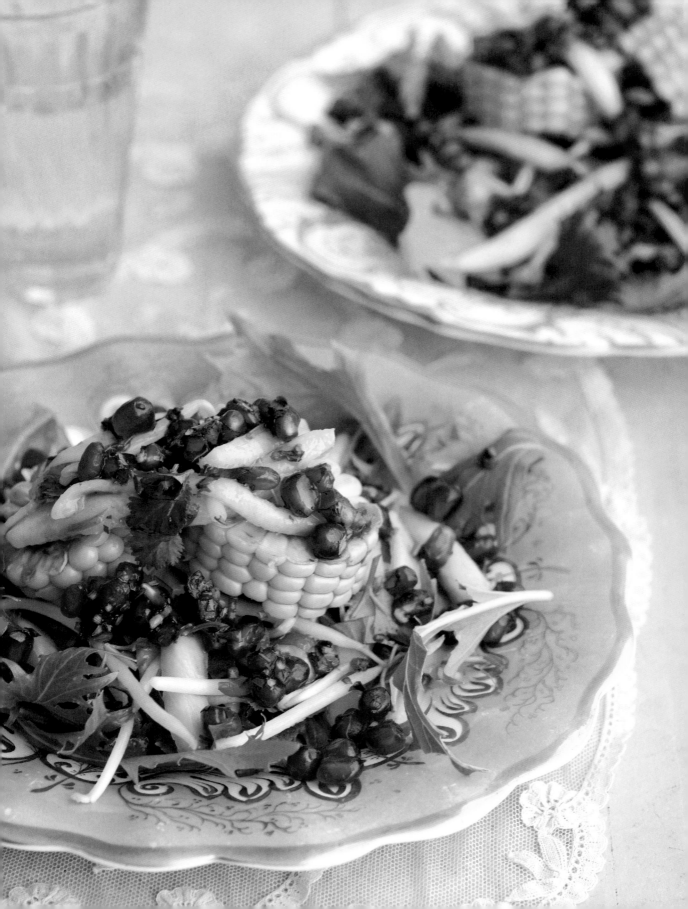

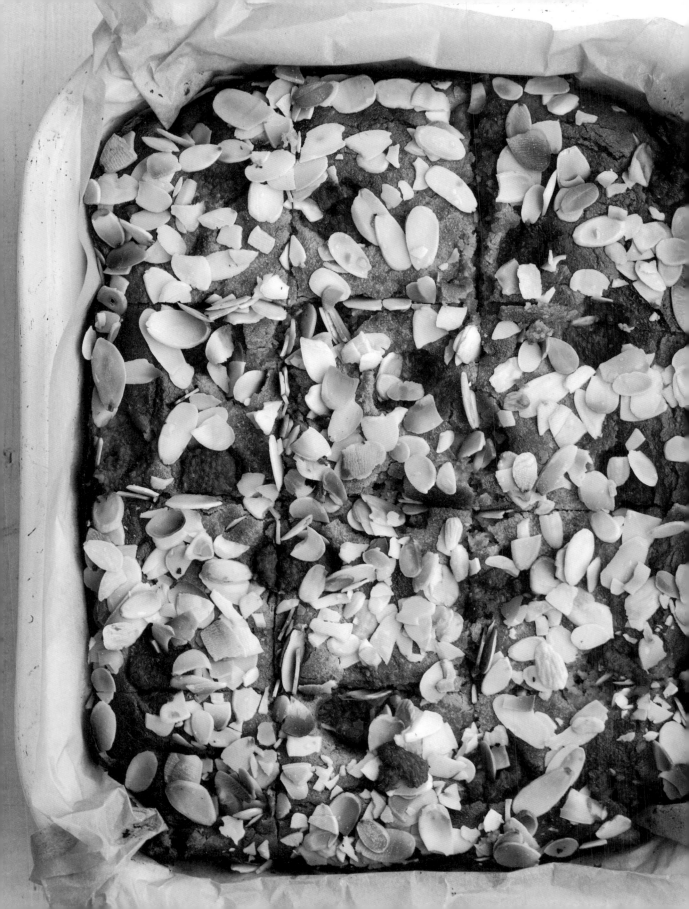

ALMOND BERRY CAKE

This is a staple sweet treat in my home—really quick to make if you have a sweet craving but also is visually stunning. The ground almonds make it a protein-rich cake, which is a welcome bonus for us vegetarians. This could be the best healthiest dessert you have ever had.

serves 9 to 12

1⅔ cups raspberries

½ cup water

2 tsp vanilla extract

4 eggs

scant ¼ cup agave syrup

¾ cup vegan butter

3⅓ cups ground almonds

1 tsp baking powder

scant ½ cup raw slivered almonds, to decorate

2¾ cups blackberries, to serve

Preheat the oven to 350°F, and line a 10-inch brownie pan with parchment paper.

Place the raspberries in a pan with the water and vanilla extract, bring to a gentle simmer over medium heat for 7 to 8 minutes. Then blend till smooth (use a whisk if you don't have a blender), set aside in a bowl, and leave to cool.

Whisk the eggs and agave together in a bowl.

In a separate bowl, mix the butter and the ground almonds together. Then add the egg mixture into the almond mix, followed by the baking powder and the raspberry purée.

Pour the cake batter into the prepared pan, scatter the slivered almonds on top, and then bake in a preheated oven for 15 minutes.

Meanwhile, gather together the blackberries and a piece of foil large enough to cover the cake. Then, as quickly as you can, take the cake out of the oven, pop the blackberries on top of the half-baked cake, re-cover with the foil, and put back into the oven for 20 minutes.

After 20 minutes test the cake—if a knife inserted into the center comes out clean, it is ready. If not, bake for another 5 minutes and test again. Remove from the oven, cool in the pan for 10 to 15 minutes, transfer to a wire rack to cool, then slice and enjoy!

TASH'S TIPS

Such a simple cake to make, you will look like a pro when it comes out of the oven. You could try different flavors— just substitute the amount of berries for another fruit compôte. Try plums for an autumnal feel.

NUTRITIONAL NUGGET

Almonds are the most alkaline of the nuts, with abundant magnesium to soothe and calm the mind. Blanched almonds have their phytate-binding skins removed so offer far better nutritional value.

BITES

BEET AND SPINACH BURGERS

How colorful are these burgers? They are super-easy to make and, if you like, you can create them bigger and serve them as a whole dish with a salad or even some sweet potato wedges for the full-on "burger and fries" effect.

makes 12 to 14 small burgers or 4 large

scant 1 cup raw quinoa

1 tbsp bouillon powder

9 oz baby spinach leaves or 7 oz boiled beet

3 tbsp sunflower oil, plus more for cooking

1 clove garlic

a pinch of Himalayan pink salt

For this recipe, you need quinoa that is really sticky, a bit like the texture of sticky rice. Cook your quinoa in twice the amount of water to grain—and, in fact, you want to overcook it. Cook the quinoa with the bouillon powder over medium heat for 20 minutes, turn off the heat and then leave it to sit in the pan with the lid on to steam, to get that sticky texture you are after, which will help to bind the burgers together without using a flour.

Meanwhile, boil some water and pour it over the spinach leaves in a strainer and leave to drain. Once drained, squeeze out the excess water and transfer to a blender with the oil and the garlic and blend till smooth. (If you want to make the beet version, swap the spinach for beet purée. To make this, blend the boiled beet and blend with the same amount of garlic, oil, and salt, then follow the steps below.)

Once the quinoa is cool enough to handle add in the spinach purée a little at a time (remember, you can't take it away). Once incorporated and still sticky you can form the mixture into burgers around the size of your palm. If they are not sticking together, you could add some oat flour a tablespoon at a time. (Make oat flour by whizzing a handful of oats in a high-speed blender.)

Preheat the oven to 350°F.

In a skillet heat 3 tablespoons of sunflower oil; you could use coconut oil instead if you prefer. Cook each burger for 2 to 3 minutes on each side, until golden. Transfer to a baking sheet and bake in the preheated oven for another 10 minutes, or until they are piping hot all the way through. Serve with Tahini Dressing (see page 82).

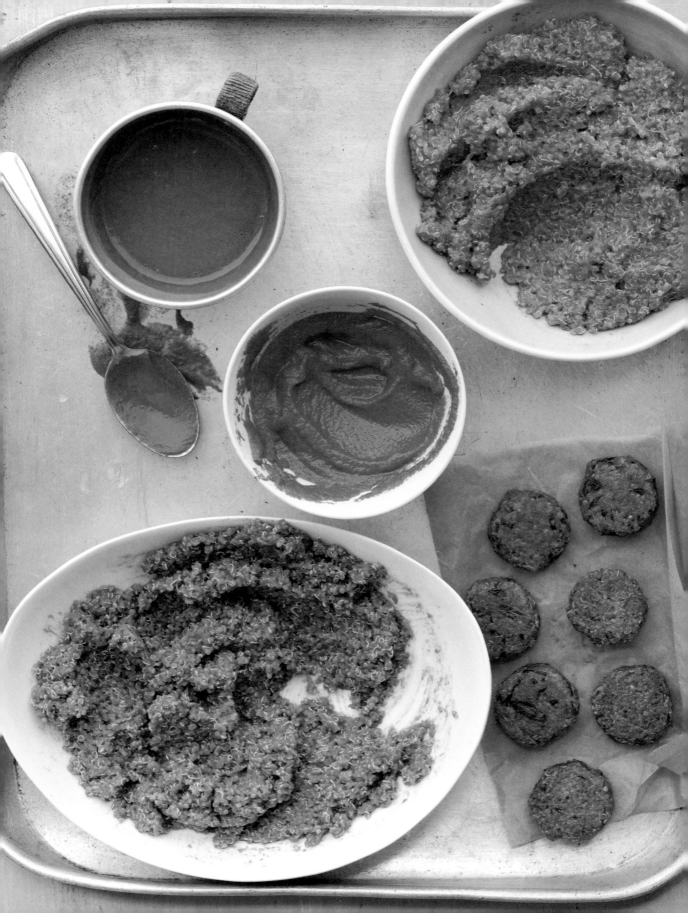

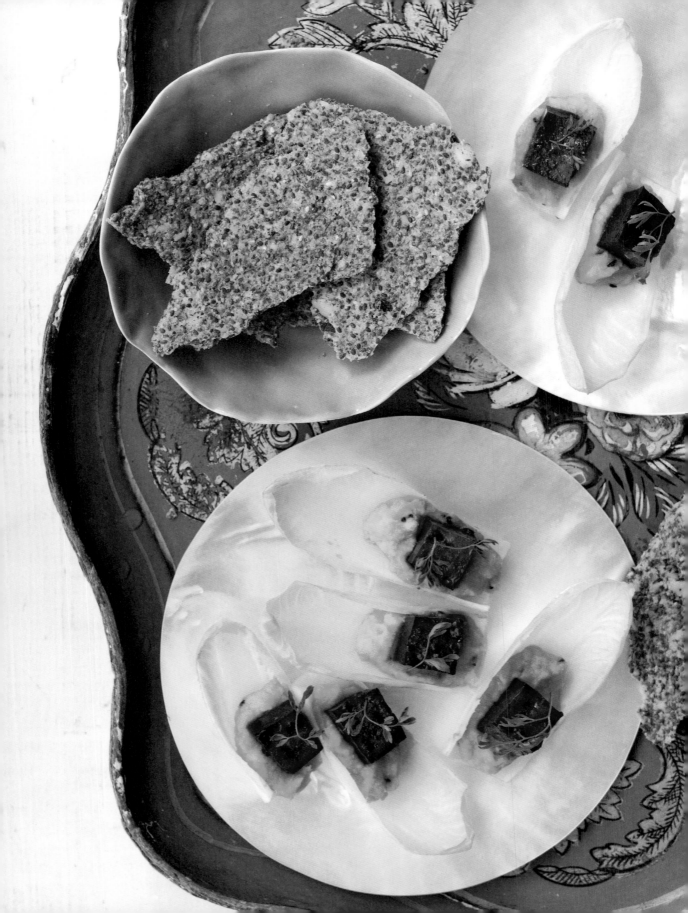

MARINATED TOFU AND ENDIVE BITES

Serve these delicate-looking bites as a pre-dinner appetizer. You could also serve these ingredients in a different way and turn it into a salad. Why not have a go at both?

makes 15 bites

4 tsp agave syrup

2 tsp tamari

2 tbsp sesame oil

3 oz plain tofu, cut into ½-in cubes

14 oz butternut squash, peeled and chopped into ¾-in chunks

1 tsp sunflower oil, plus 1 tbsp for frying

¼ tsp Himalayan pink salt

¼ tsp black onion seeds

3 tbsp sweet miso

a squeeze of lemon (¼ lemon)

⅛ tbsp black onion seeds

2 heads of endive

3 tbsp cilantro, chopped

Preheat the oven to 350°F.

In a small bowl make the marinade by mixing together the agave, tamari, and half the sesame oil, then put the cubed tofu in it to marinate for 30 minutes.

Toss the butternut chunks in 1 teaspoon of the sunflower oil with the salt and black onion seeds. Roast in the preheated oven for 15 minutes. Remove from the oven and set aside to cool.

When the roasted butternut has cooled, transfer to a blender or food processor along with the sweet miso, the rest of the sesame oil, the lemon juice, and the ⅛ tablespoon of black onion seeds and whiz until smooth. Set aside.

Break off the endive leaves one by one, and place them in a colander. Rinse them under the faucet and set aside on a dishtowel to drip dry.

Heat a tablespoon of sunflower oil in a skillet over medium heat. Put the marinated tofu in the pan, along with the remaining marinade. The tofu needs to cook and be turned until the marinade starts to caramelize and become sticky. Make sure it doesn't burn and take it off the heat once all the liquid has gone.

Line up the endive leaves on a serving board. Put a ½ tablespoon of the squash purée onto the leaf, followed by a piece of tofu, and then garnish with fresh cilantro.

BRAZIL NUT RAW CRACKERS

These are a great alternative to crackers and, if you have time to make them, they are so rewarding. Perfect to enjoy as a protein afternoon snack, with a dip, or for a crunchy partner to the tofu bites.

½ cup chia seeds

½ cup water

1 cup raw brazil nuts

a handful of sage leaves

3 tbsp olive oil

a pinch of black pepper

1 clove garlic, grated

1 tsp Celtic sea salt

In a high-speed blender (or coffee grinder) grind half the chia seeds. Soak the ground and whole seeds in the water for 15 minutes. Then, drain and set aside. Preheat the dehydrator to 104°F. In a food processor or blender, blend the brazil nuts and half the sage with the olive oil, pepper, grated garlic, and salt. Pulse a few times to break down the brazil nuts for a hearty textured cracker, or process until fine for a thinner cracker. Then, mix into the soaked chia seeds mixture and roughly chop the remaining sage and mix in.

Spread to a thickness of ¼ inch on a dehydrator tray, then pop in the dehydrator for 10 hours. See page 84 if you don't have a dehydrator.

MINI SUSHI ROLLS

A tray of these gorgeous little rolls makes a great appetizer or a pre-dinner bite and will help keep your guests' bellies from rumbling. They do take a little practice to get them into a tight roll, but as they say practice makes perfect, so keep rolling!

♥ ♥ ♥

makes 24 rolls

scant ¼ cup red or white quinoa

1 cup brown sushi rice

4 tbsp brown rice vinegar

¼ tsp apple cider vinegar

1 tbsp mirin

2 tbsp water

1 tsp agave syrup

1 tsp Himalayan pink salt

4 sheets of nori seaweed

tamari and wasabi, to serve

Ideas for sushi roll fillings:

daikon, grated or sliced

mixed lettuce leaves and/or sliced cucumber

thinly sliced green beans

cilantro or flat-leaf parsley

grated carrot

sliced avocado

toasted white sesame seeds

toasted sunflower seeds

Cook the quinoa and brown sushi rice separately according to the package instructions and set aside.

Meanwhile, stir the vinegars, mirin, water, agave syrup, and salt together in a bowl until fully mixed. Set aside.

Transfer the rice and quinoa into a large bowl and then gently mix the vinegar mixture into the rice, spreading the grains out a little as you mix to help dry and cool the rice and quinoa. Let the rice mixture cool until it's warm, around 10 minutes of stirring and fanning.

Place a nori sheet onto a bamboo sushi mat. With wet fingers, lightly press the rice to cover around a quarter of a nori sheet in an even layer, leaving around ½ inch uncovered at the top of the sheet. Then—time to get creative—place whichever filling ingredients you're using in a line across the bottom of the rice. (Make sure you don't put too much filling in as you will find it hard to roll the parcel up and they may well spill out sideways when you cut them.)

Pick up the edge of the bamboo rolling mat, fold the bottom edge of the mat up, enclosing the filling, and tightly roll the sushi into a thick cylinder. Once the sushi is rolled, wrap it in the mat and give it a gentle squeeze to compact it tightly.

Unwrap the rolling mat, and cut the sushi cylinder into six pieces to serve; repeat with the remaining ingredients to make three more rolls.

Serve with tamari sauce and wasabi for your guests to dip into as they wish.

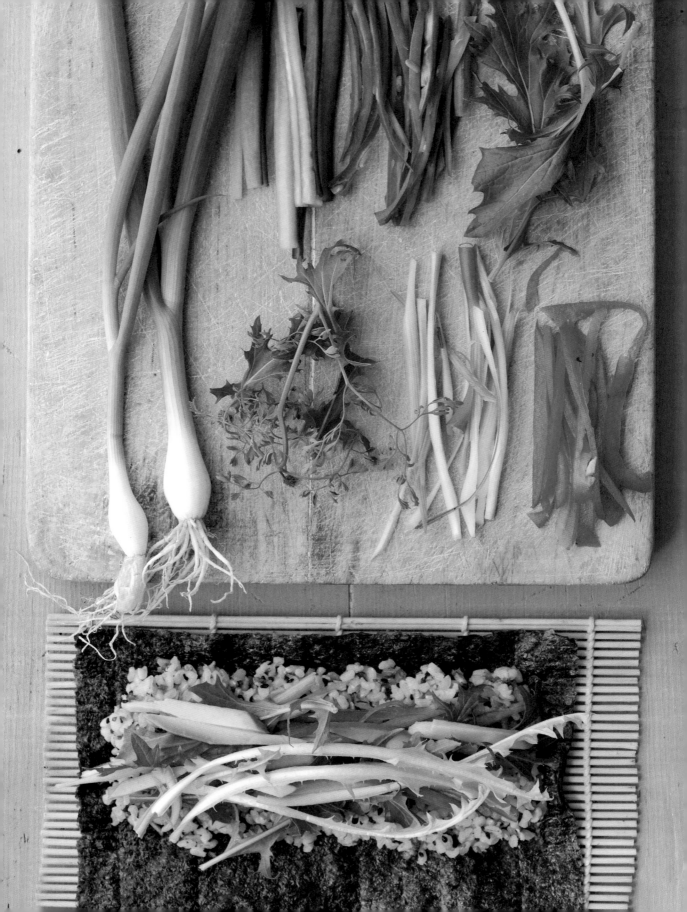

DINNER FOR 2 OR 12

ROASTED TOMATO AND SPINACH TART

All I can say about this recipe is you just have to try it! Once you've tasted it, it's sure to become a regular feature in your cooking repertoire.

serves 6

For the crust:
2¼ cups ground almonds
2 sprigs rosemary
4 tbsp sunflower oil
½ tsp caraway seeds
a pinch of Himalayan pink salt
1 tbsp water
generous ¾ cup raw pumpkin seeds
⅓ cup raw sunflower seeds

For the topping:
1 lb 2 oz tomatoes
2 cloves garlic
4 tbsp olive oil, plus 1 tsp
1 tbsp picked thyme leaves, plus a few sprigs
½ tsp Himalayan pink salt
¼ tsp cracked black pepper
2 tbsp balsamic vinegar
14 oz spinach leaves
⅔ cup hard goat's cheese, grated

Preheat the oven to 325°F and line a 7½-inch tart or cake pan with parchment paper. You'll also need a baking sheet lined with parchment paper.

Pulse the ground almonds, rosemary, sunflower oil, caraway seeds, salt, water, and half the pumpkin seeds until smooth and set aside.

Then pulse the rest of the pumpkin seeds and the sunflower seeds, but only for a few seconds to ensure you are keeping some texture for the crust.

Mix the seeds into the ground almond mixture. Combine thoroughly until the mixture starts to come together. Press it into the prepared pan and bake for 25 minutes until golden.

Meanwhile, quarter the tomatoes and finely chop the garlic. In a large bowl, make a marinade from 4 tablespoons of the olive oil, the thyme, salt, pepper, and vinegar and add in the garlic. Toss the tomatoes in the marinade then tip out onto a baking sheet and roast for 8 minutes. Remove from the oven and set aside.

Meanwhile, wilt the spinach by pouring boiling hot water over it in a colander and then cool it down by running cold water over it over the sink. Once cooled, squeeze out all the excess water and finely chop or blitz the spinach with a teaspoon of olive oil.

Remove the crust from the oven and scatter the spinach over the base of the tart, top with the roasted tomatoes, and then sprinkle over the grated goat's cheese.

Garnish with a few sprigs of thyme and then bake for another 15 minutes, until the cheese has melted. Serve straightaway and enjoy.

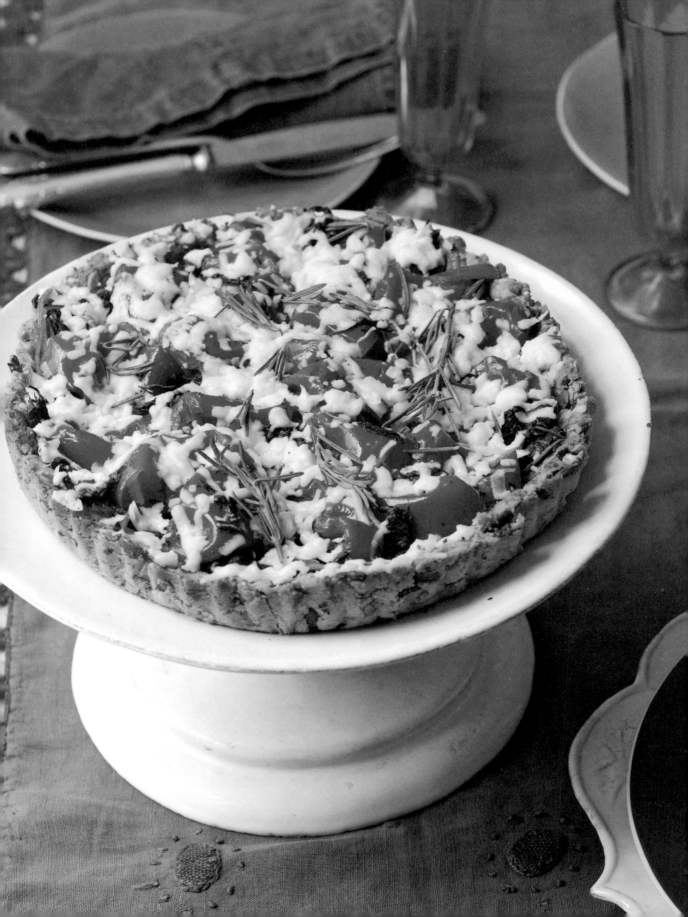

ROASTED EGGPLANT AND MANGO SALSA WITH BLACK RICE NOODLES

In this dish the contrast of colors is simply stunning and I love to serve it up to friends or family. If you can't get black rice noodles, don't worry, you can use normal rice noodles instead.

serves 4

2 eggplant, roughly cut into ¾-in cubes

3 tbsp sunflower oil

1 red onion, thinly sliced

½ tsp ground ginger

½ tsp ground coriander

a pinch of Himalayan pink salt

9 oz black rice noodles

4 tsp sesame oil

1 large mango, cut into ½-in cubes

1¼ cups cilantro, chopped

finely grated zest of 1 lemon

1 tsp black onion seeds

raw sesame seeds, to garnish

½-in chili, sliced at an angle, to garnish

Preheat the oven to 325°F and line a baking sheet with parchment paper.

In a large bowl, toss the eggplant with the sunflower oil, red onion, ground ginger, ground coriander, and salt. Place onto the prepared baking sheet and roast for 20 minutes.

Meanwhile, in a large pan of boiling water, cook the black rice noodles and keep stirring them to ensure they don't stick to each other. When cooked, refresh immediately (drain and plunge into cold water) and pour the sesame oil over them to keep them from sticking to each other. Gluten-free noodles can be tricky!

Once the eggplant is roasted, remove from the oven and let cool.

In another bowl, mix the mango cubes with the chopped cilantro, lemon zest, and black onion seeds. Mix this "mango salsa" with the roasted eggplant. Split the mixture, and gently mix half of it into the noodles.

Portion the noodles into four bowls and top with the rest of the salsa mixture along with a sprinkling of sesame seeds and fresh chili for color. It's also great with some Tahini Dressing swirled on top (see page 82).

NUTRITIONAL NUGGET

Black rice is incredibly rich in minerals, being the most dense of all the rices. Manganese and calcium support bone health, while zinc aids the immune system, as well as the rice being a source of soluble fiber.

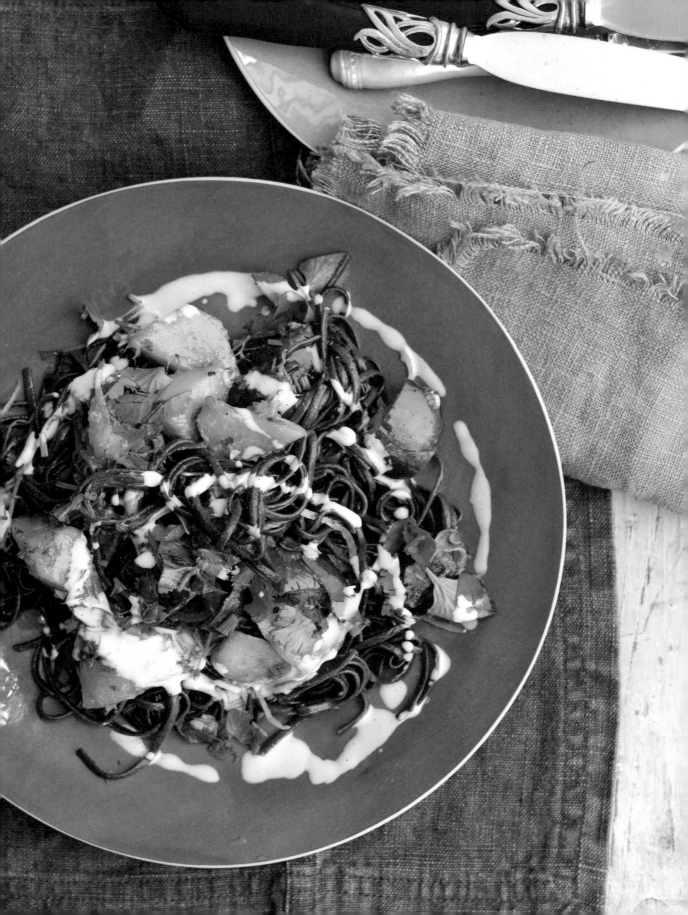

SPICED DHAL

*This is one of my favorite weekend feasts—it's
simple, filling, and delicious—it even keeps the most
ravenous meat-eaters happy. And you can rustle up
some Buckwheat Flatbreads (see page 219) while
the dhal is cooking!*

serves 4

5 cardamom pods

¼ tsp dried chili flakes (optional)

4–5 whole black peppercorns

1 tsp coriander seeds

1 tsp ground cumin

1 tsp ground cinnamon

1 tbsp garam masala

1 tsp turmeric

a thumb-sized knob of ginger root

2 cloves garlic

½ red chili

2 oz cilantro

1 tsp mixed herbs

a pinch of Himalayan pink salt

3 tbsp sunflower oil

2 tbsp water

2 white onions, finely chopped

1¼ cups red split lentils

1¼ cups mint, chopped

⅓ cup soy yogurt

a squeeze of lemon

Toast the cardamom, dried chili flakes, whole black
peppercorns, and coriander seeds in a dry skillet
over medium heat for 1 to 2 minutes.

Once toasted, put into the blender along with all the
spices, fresh ginger, garlic, chili, herbs, and a pinch
of salt. Blend with 2 tablespoons of sunflower oil
and 2 tablespoons of water to create a paste.

Heat 1 tablespoon of sunflower oil in a large skillet
and sauté the onions over medium heat. Just
before the onions become translucent add the
spice paste and cook for a good 15 minutes,
constantly adding splashes of cool water (around
1 tablespoon at a time) to the pan to keep the
temperature down and keep the paste from
sticking to the bottom of the pan.

Add the red lentils to the pan and give them a good
stir to coat them in the paste. Then pour 2½ cups of
water into the pan, covering the lentils. Allow it to
cook on a gentle heat for another 20 minutes. Give
it the occasional stir to make sure the lentils are
not sticking to the bottom of the pan; if at this point
the lentils have absorbed all the water add another
1 cup or however much of that you need. Once the
lentils have tripled in size and absorbed most of the
water take the pan off the heat and leave it to cool
for 10 minutes before serving.

Serve with some chopped fresh mint mixed into
the soy yogurt along with a squeeze of lemon and
with the Buckwheat Flatbreads (see page 219).

Mango chutney

¼ red onion

¼-in piece of ginger root

1 small fresh mango

finely grated zest of 1 lime

a pinch of chili flakes

Finely dice the onion and put in a bowl, and grate
the ginger over the top.

Dice the mango and put half in with the onion and
ginger and blend the other half into a purée—this
will be the "sauce" that holds the chutney together.

Add the purée to the rest of the ingredients, mix
well, and season to taste with the lime zest and a
tiny pinch of chili flakes.

NUTRITIONAL NUGGET
Red split lentils are one of the most
prominently used sources of protein
in Asian cooking, with the slow-
release carbohydrate content making
them both a nourishing and an
energizing food.

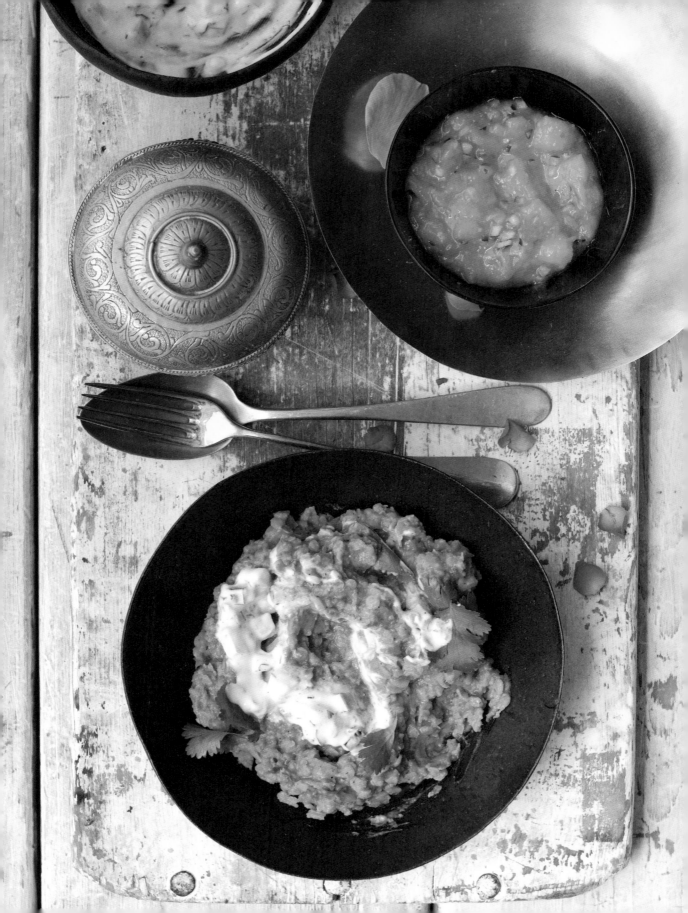

SPINACH PEARL BARLEY "RISOTTO"

This is a perfect simple dinner to make and, once you've got the hang of the technique, it's fun to play around with new flavors—stir in different purées toward the end of the cooking time. Do bear in mind that pearl barley has gluten so is no good for those with a gluten allergy, but you can substitute brown risotto rice instead.

serves 4

3 tbsp bouillon powder

3½ cups boiling water

2 small red onions

2 cloves garlic

3 tbsp sunflower oil

scant 1 cup pearl barley

7 oz baby spinach leaves or 4 cooked beets

a pinch of Himalayan pink salt

2 oz cilantro

finely grated zest of 1 lemon

juice of ½ lemon

Add the bouillon powder to the boiling water to make a vegetable stock and stir until all the powder has dissolved. Set aside.

Finely chop the onions and one of the cloves of garlic and sauté in a large pan with 2 tablespoons of sunflower oil over medium heat. Add the pearl barely and stir it around the pan for a minute before slowly adding the stock. The barley should start absorbing the liquid (just as the rice in a risotto would).

When you have used around half the stock and the barley has absorbed most of the liquid, pour the remaining stock into the pan and allow the barley to cook for another 15 minutes over medium heat. Be sure to keep an eye on the barley and stir constantly to make sure it doesn't stick to the bottom of the pan. This will also create the classic creaminess of a risotto.

Meanwhile, put the baby spinach or beets, whichever you prefer, into a blender with a pinch of salt and the remaining sunflower oil and clove of garlic. Whiz into a smooth purée.

When the barley is cooked and all the liquid has been absorbed, add the purée into the "risotto," cook for another 3 minutes, then turn off the heat.

Roughly chop the cilantro and add to the risotto along with the lemon zest and juice, and serve straightaway.

♥♥ Pina Nutada

This twist on the traditional Pina Colada really is a knock out creamy concoction! Whether you choose to have it with, or without the vodka, this high-protein drink gives you plenty of energy, as well as feeding your skin from within from all the essential fats found in the almonds.

MAKES 4 SMALL OR 2 LARGE GLASSES

generous 2 cups unsweetened almond milk
  (homemade or from a carton)

a pinch of cinnamon

a pinch of nutmeg, grated

3 drops vanilla extract (optional, for added
  sweetness)

4 shots vodka (quinoa vodka is best)

a pinch of ground cumin, to serve over the top
  (optional)

Mix all the ingredients in a blender, and chill before serving over crushed ice. The pinch of cumin on top "knocks" the sweetness. Leave out vodka and cumin for the kids—they'll love it, too.

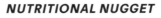

NUTRITIONAL NUGGET

This dish offers a brilliant way to pack in a lot of iron-rich spinach when you aren't green juicing. The fiber in spinach is essential to maintain a healthy digestive system.

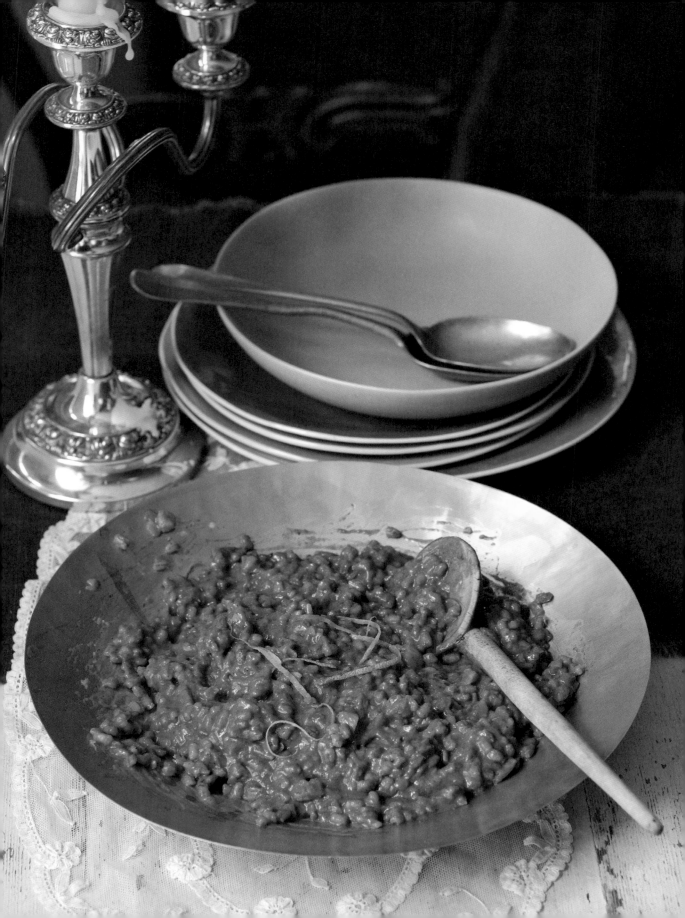

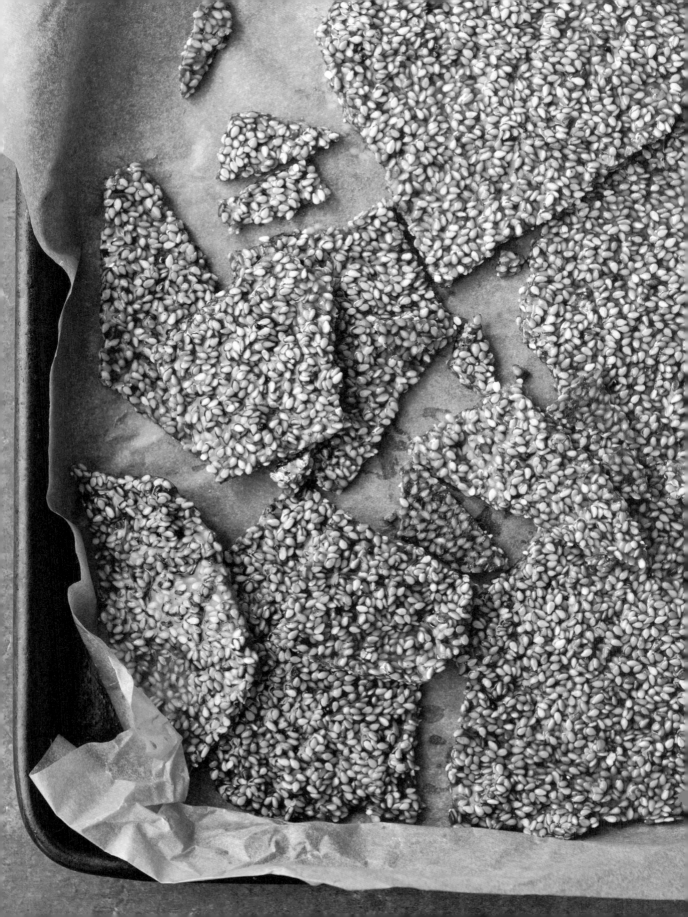

SESAME BRITTLE

This treat is indulgence at its best—the brittle can be kept in the freezer and will last for a good two months, if you don't gobble it up sooner. It is fantastic broken over ice cream (see page 222), used in a salad for an extra sweet and salty crunch, or on its own as a delightful treat.

makes a whole tray

½ cup coconut palm sugar

scant ½ cup agave syrup

6 tbsp vegan butter

½ tsp vanilla extract

¼ tsp baking soda

¼ tsp Himalayan pink salt

⅛ tsp cayenne pepper (optional)

1⅓ cups raw sesame seeds

Line a baking sheet with parchment paper and set aside.

Place a nonstick pan over medium heat and add the coconut palm sugar and agave. Stir with a wooden spoon to help the sugars dissolve. Once all the coconut palm sugar has dissolved, add all the other ingredients apart from the sesame seeds (the cayenne pepper gives the brittle a good "kick," so add less, or none, if you don't want it too spicy).

Turn the temperature up to high heat for 5 minutes or so, bringing the mixture to a rapid boil. Be careful as it is extremely hot! Once it has reached boiling point, let the mixture bubble for another 2 minutes and then take it off the heat. Quickly stir in the sesame seeds at this point.

Pour the mixture onto the prepared baking sheet and freeze for 2 hours or overnight. Keep in the freezer until you want to serve it, whichever way you choose.

TASH'S TIPS

This comes with a warning...only have a little bit as a treat! Make sure you bring it to a boil as it will not set properly otherwise.

NUTRITIONAL NUGGET

Sesame seeds are packed with selenium, which is now sadly lacking in our soil, due to over-farming. Selenium is required for immunity, skin repair, and better brain function, as well as boosting metabolism.

LEMONGRASS AND ROSE WATER PANNACOTTA

If you want a showstopper of a dessert then this is the one. As well as being utterly mouthwatering, this guilt-free custard can last around three days in the refrigerator; so, if you have any left over (which I doubt you will, but here's hoping) you can always dig in later in the week to satisfy a sweet craving.

makes 4

1¾ cups coconut milk

scant ¼ cup rice milk

1 lemongrass, cut lengthwise down the middle
   for infusing

scant ¼ cup xylitol

½ vanilla bean, split and scraped, or 2 tsp
   vanilla extract

2 tsp agar agar

1¼ tsp rose water

rose petals, for decoration

You'll need four 3-inch ramekins or molds, or you could use glass cups.

Pour the coconut milk and rice milk into a pan and add the lemongrass. Then place the pan over medium heat and bring it to a gentle simmer for 5 minutes. Next, add the xylitol and vanilla seeds (or extract) and allow it to simmer for another 5 minutes.

Remove the lemongrass and discard. Then add the agar agar. Stir or whisk the mixture until the agar agar has completely dissolved.

Take the pan off the heat, add the rose water, and then strain the mixture through a strainer to ensure a smooth texture. Pour the strained mixture into four molds or ramekins and allow them to set in the refrigerator for 3 hours.

Put some rose petals in the freezer for 2 hours, to decorate.

Turn out onto individual plates (simply invert onto a plate and tap the bottom of the mold until it flumps out; see also my tip below) and decorate with frosted rose petals.

TASH'S TIPS
These little beauties are delicate when still in the cup or mold. I gently push mine with a finger around the edges so that it starts to release the suction and moves slightly within the cup or mold. Then, it's just a case of putting a plate on top, inverting it, and tapping the bottom to let it slip out.

NUTRITIONAL NUGGET
Lemongrass is used extensively in Asia for its anti-bacterial and anti-viral cleansing properties. This recipe infuses its delicate flavor, while adding coconut milk, which is protein-rich and immune-boosting.

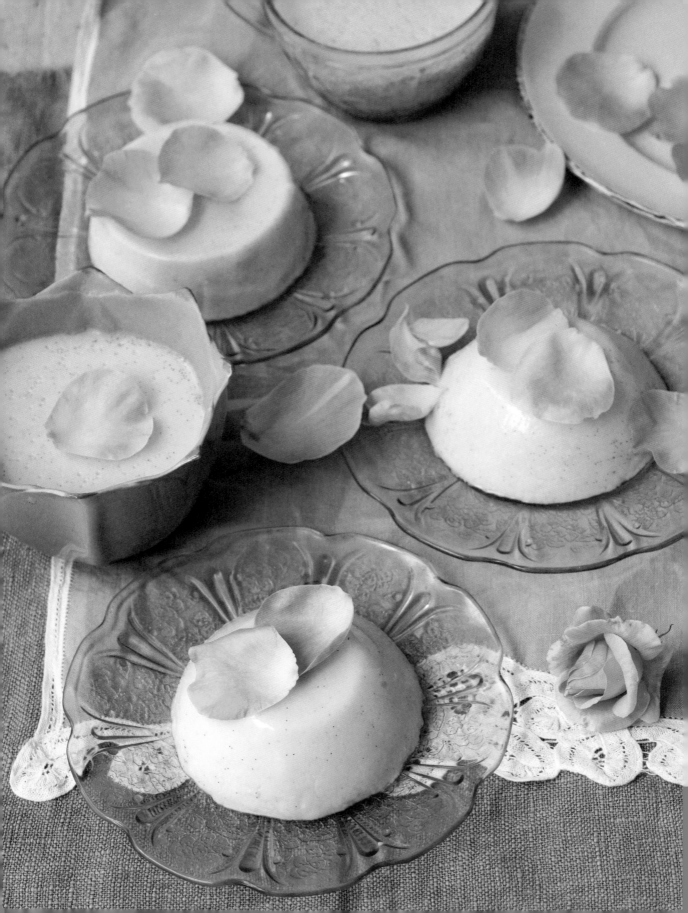

FIXERS AND BOOSTERS

Life is not always plain sailing, so it's good to know there's a wealth of healing juices and drinks to help get you back on your feet again. Whether you're feeling tired all the time, a bit blue, or need to beat a cold or bout of flu, each recipe is designed to contain exactly the nutrients your body needs to heal itself again.

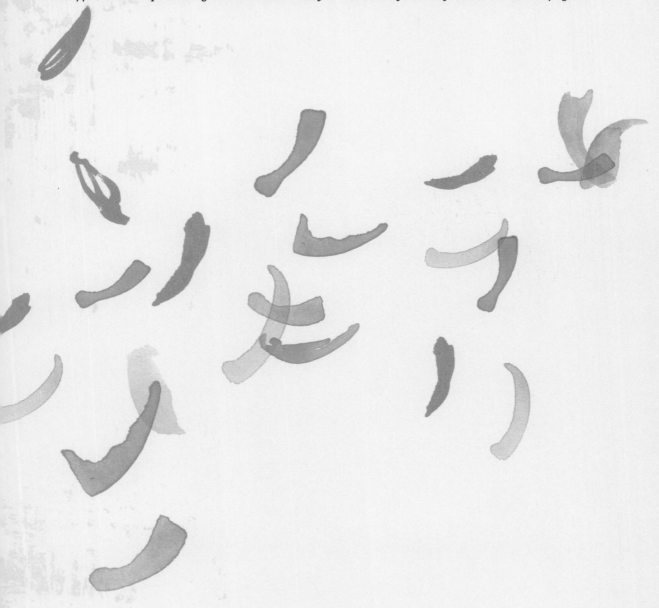

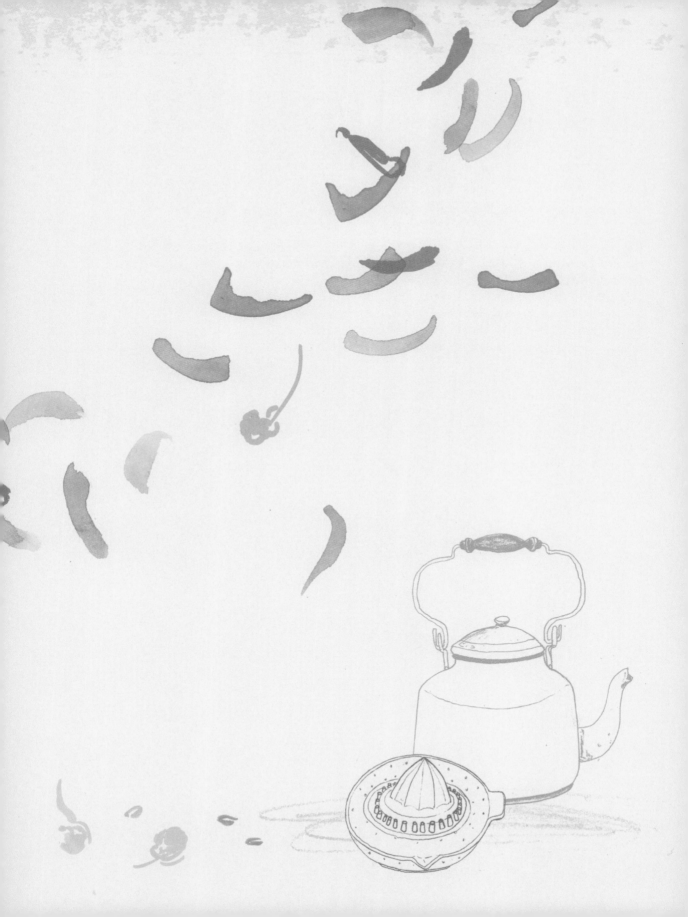

BREAK-UP CURE

HOT CHOCOLATE WITH CASHEW

There is nothing better to turn to when we are a bit down in the dumps than a good hot chocolate. This warming mug of comfort will lift your mood because the cashews that we have put into it are high in niacin—a mood enhancer. Did you know that a handful of cashews is the equivalent of a dose of Prozac? So, after this warming chocolatey delight there will be no more tears.

serves 2

generous 2 cups dairy-free coconut milk

2 heaping tbsp raw cacao powder

1 handful raw cashew nuts

2 tbsp sugar substitute (brown rice syrup or
　agave syrup)

Whiz all the ingredients together in a blender until smooth.

Transfer to a pan and warm up to the desired temperature over low heat.

Pour into mugs and slip away into a healthy chocolate coma. If you'd like an added extra, swirl some dairy-free cream (see Raw Banoffee Pie, page 171) on top. Yum!

TASH'S TIPS
If you like your hot chocolate on the watery side, you can simply leave out the cashews and add 4 tablespoons or so of water.

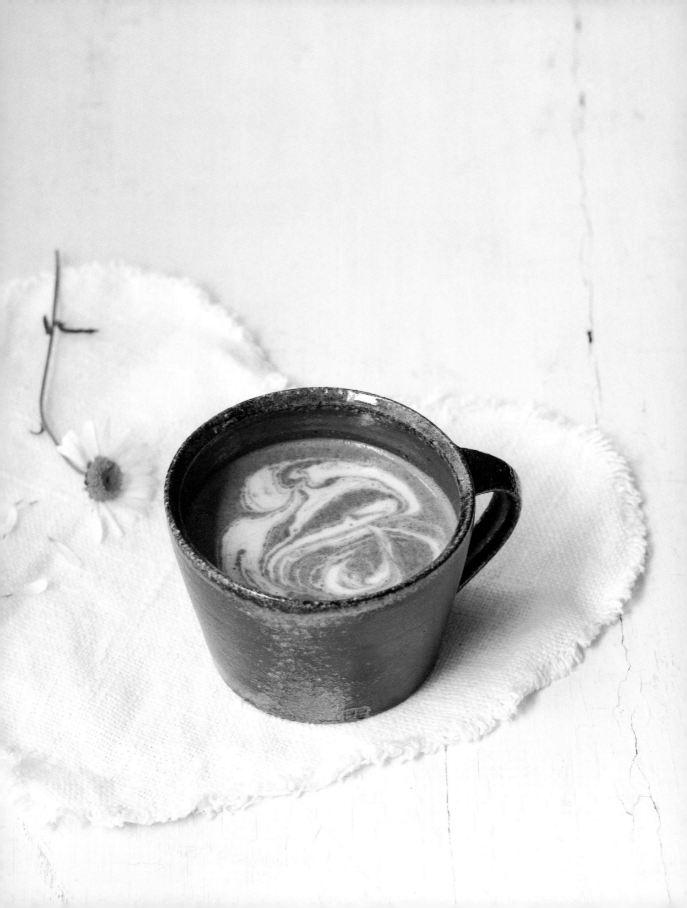

TEAS AND TISANES

Break-Up Cure Tea—Rosebud, Chamomile, and Cinnamon

This combination of spices and flowers hits a relaxing note. Both cinnamon and nutmeg are calming (as well as being anti-inflammatory). Chamomile is relaxing and a great digestive herb (helping to expel excess gas in the system), while rosebuds induce feelings of relaxation.

2 tsp dried rosebuds
2 chamomile flowers (dried or fresh)
small stick of cinnamon
a pinch of grated nutmeg
generous 2 cups just-boiled water

Add just-boiled water to the herbs, spices, and tea leaves and allow them to infuse for 10 to 12 minutes before serving. Strain through muslin or a tea strainer and serve immediately.

Flat Tummy Tea—Nettle, Fennel, Slippery Elm, and Peppermint

Nettle and fennel are natural diuretics (allowing the body to expel any retained water), while slippery elm calms any intestinal inflammation. Peppermint is widely known for its powers of aiding digestion.

1 bag each of the following teas: nettle, fennel, and peppermint
a pinch of slippery elm tea leaves or powder
generous 2 cups just-boiled water

Infuse all the tea bags, together with the slippery elm leaves or powder, in just-boiled water for 15 minutes before serving. Strain through muslin or a tea strainer and serve immediately. Alternatively, let cool and store in the refrigerator—sip throughout the day, especially after meals, for optimum effects.

Fatigue Fighter Tea—Yerba Mate, White Tea, and Rosemary

Yerba mate is an ancient tea from the Incas (of South America); made from leaves of a holly tree, the Incas used this tea for enhancing vigor. Rosemary is a highly stimulating herb and gives this tea a pick-me-up quality; but it should be used in moderation to prevent palpitations. White tea is known to stimulate the immune system and energy production, as well as being cleansing and weight lowering.

1 tsp yerba mate
½ tsp pure white tea leaves
1 small sprig rosemary
generous 2 cups just-boiled water

Add just-boiled water to the herbs, spices, and tea leaves and allow them to infuse for 10 minutes before serving. Strain through muslin or a tea strainer and serve immediately. This tea can also be served chilled, but do not allow the leaves to stand for longer than 10 minutes before straining, as they will become too bitter.

Flu Fix Tisane—Star Anise, Ginger, and Lemon

Star anise stimulates the immune system greatly, as does fresh ginger root, thereby helping your body fight germs more effectively. In addition, the oil from the lemon zest and lemon juice are rich in vitamin C, which boosts the body's natural defenses.

2 star anise
a thumbful of fresh ginger root, grated roughly
finely grated zest and juice of ½ lemon
generous 2 cups just-boiled water

Allow all the ingredients to steep in just-boiled water for 15 to 20 minutes before drinking. Add extra water throughout the day and sip regularly.

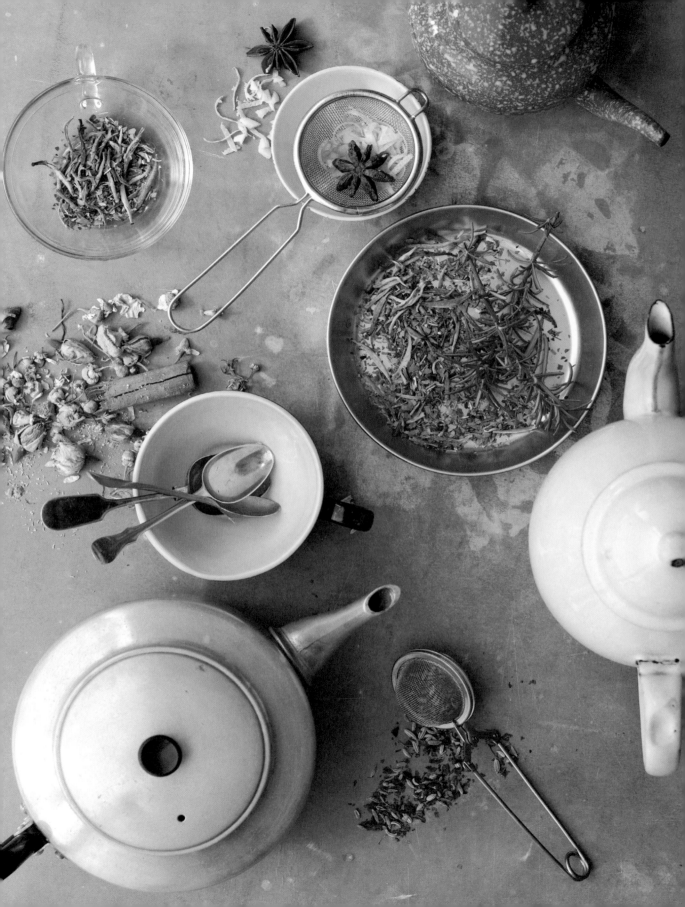

FLU FIX

CARROT AND CARAWAY SOUP

If you are coming down with a cold, there's nothing more comforting than a wonderfully warming soup to nurse you back to health. This delicious soup also works as a perfect appetizer for a dinner party.

serves 4

1 tbsp bouillon powder

5 cups boiling water

2 tbsp sunflower oil

1 large white onion, finely chopped

2 cloves garlic, finely chopped

1 tsp ground cumin

1 tbsp caraway seeds

2¼ lb carrots, peeled and chopped into chunks

2 star anise

½ cup cilantro, roughly chopped

1 tbsp umeboshi plum purée

Add the bouillon powder to the boiling water to make a vegetable stock and stir until all the powder has dissolved. Set aside.

Gently heat the sunflower oil in a pan and sauté the onion and garlic. Sprinkle in the cumin and stir through. Add the caraway seeds to the pan and add small splashes (1–2 tablespoons) of cool water to the pan to bring the temperature down. Once the onions are translucent add the carrots.

Next, add the vegetable stock and the star anise— these float on the surface of the soup and as they bob around they infuse the liquid with lovely flavors. Allow the pan to simmer over gentle heat for 30 minutes.

Take the pan off the heat and transfer the contents to a blender (remove the star anise now). Whiz until smooth, adding the cilantro and umeboshi plum purée to season to taste before serving. Check the temperature of the soup—it should be hot enough, but if not pop it back in the pan and reheat. Serve piping hot.

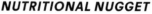

NUTRITIONAL NUGGET

Star anise has potent anti-viral properties, as does garlic. Used together, they knock out the flu virus.

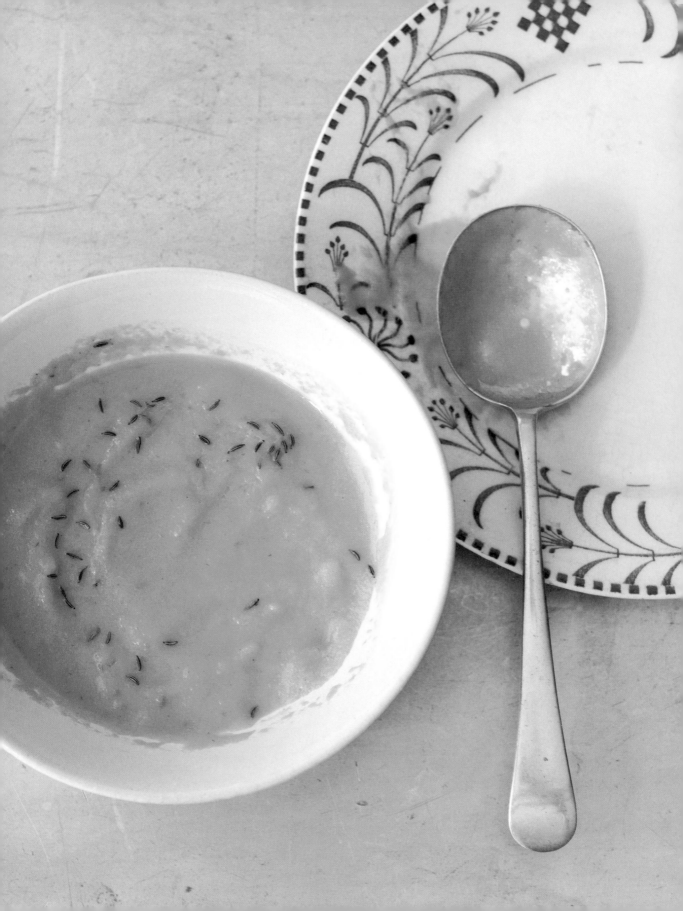

CHESTNUT AND APRICOT SOUP

This is such an earthy dish, a perfect winter warming soup to curl up on the sofa with, and it helps to boost your immune system.

serves 2

1 tbsp bouillon powder

6⅓ cups boiling water

1 tbsp sunflower oil

1 large leek (around 5¾ oz), chopped

1 clove garlic, finely chopped

2 small bay leaves

1 tsp freshly picked thyme leaves, plus sprigs
  to garnish (optional)

½ tsp ground coriander

9 oz cooked ready-to-eat chestnuts, roughly
  chopped

½ cup dried apricots, roughly chopped

Add the bouillon powder to the boiling water to make a vegetable stock and stir until all the powder has dissolved. Set aside.

Gently heat the sunflower oil in a medium-sized pan and sauté the leek and garlic. Add the bay leaves, thyme, and ground coriander to the pan and stir. When the onions are translucent, stir in the chestnuts and dried apricots. Next, add the stock and cook on a gentle simmer for 25 minutes.

Take the pan off the heat and transfer the contents to a blender (removing the bay leaves). Whiz until smooth. Check the temperature of the soup—it should be hot enough, but if not pop it back in the pan and reheat. Serve piping hot and garnish each bowl with a sprig of thyme, if you like.

NUTRITIONAL NUGGET
The beta-carotene in apricots
boosts immunity.

CELERIAC AND ORANGE SOUP

This is one of my favorite soups to make—it's so velvety and the flavors are deliciously soft. This is not only great for a flu fix but is good for combating water retention. It also makes a fab appetizer for a dinner party, too, with the beautiful zest on the top.

serves 4

1 bulb fennel (around 10½ oz), chopped into
  1-in cubes

5 tbsp sunflower oil

1 clove garlic, chopped

1 onion, chopped

1 tbsp bouillon powder

3½ cups water

6 cups celeriac (around 2 lb), chopped

1⅔ cups coconut milk

1 tbsp umeboshi plum purée

finely grated zest of 1 orange, to garnish

Preheat the oven to 325°F.

First, roast the fennel with 2 tablespoons of oil for 30 minutes. Remove from the oven and set aside.

In a pan on a high heat, add the garlic, onion, and remaining oil and sauté for 2 minutes. Dissolve the bouillon powder in scant ¼ cup of boiling water and add to the pan. Simmer for another 2 minutes over medium heat. Add 1 cup of the water and simmer for another 2 minutes.

Add the chopped celeriac and roasted fennel to the pan and cover with the remaining water. Leave to cook over medium heat for 40 minutes. Then, add the coconut milk and the umeboshi plum purée.

Transfer the contents of the pan to a blender and blend until smooth. Check the temperature of the soup—it should be hot enough, but if not pop it back in the pan and reheat. Serve piping hot with the zest of orange sprinkled over the top.

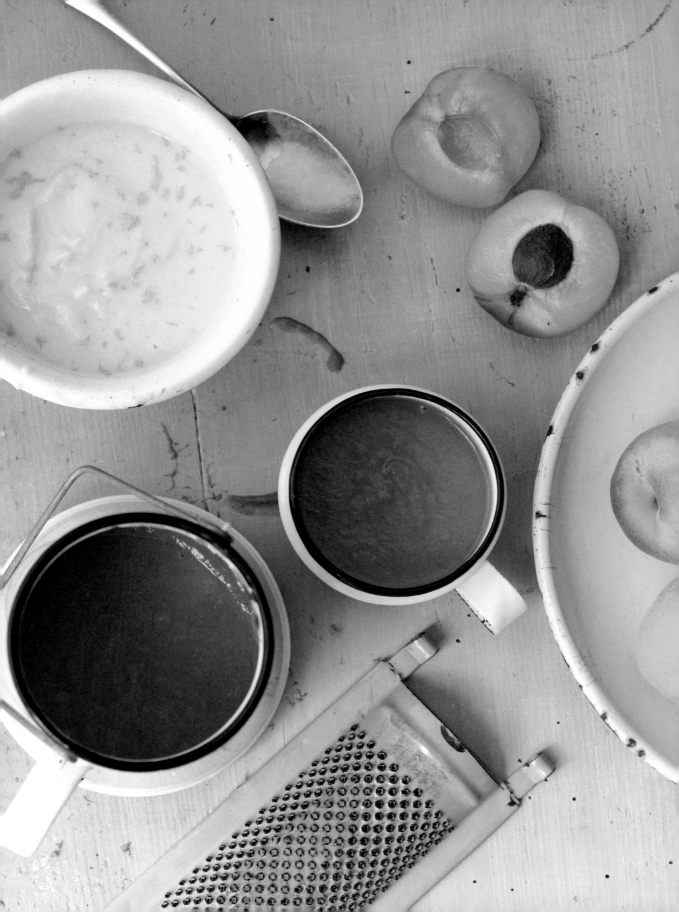

FLAT TUMMY

FENNEL AND LEEK SOUP

Fennel is one of my favorite vegetables and is great for getting rid of retained water, which many people need to do. Put your feet up and enjoy the feeling that you're getting slimmer with every spoonful!

serves 2

1 large bulb fennel (around 13 oz)

1 large leek (around 5 oz)

2 tbsp sunflower oil

¼ tsp Himalayan pink salt

1 tbsp bouillon powder

3½ cups boiling water

1 white onion, finely chopped

1 clove garlic, finely chopped

½ tsp ground fenugreek

½ tsp ground coriander

¾ oz cilantro

juice of ½ lemon

Preheat the oven to 325°F. You'll need a baking sheet.

Roughly chop up the fennel and leek, toss them in 1 tablespoon of sunflower oil and the salt, and roast in the oven for 20 minutes.

Meanwhile, add the bouillon powder to the boiling water to make a vegetable stock and stir until all the powder has dissolved. Set aside.

Heat the remaining sunflower oil in a pan over the lowest possible heat. Add the onions and garlic and sauté together with the ground spices (while the fennel and leek is roasting). Keep adding small splashes (1–2 tablespoons) of the stock to keep the pan cool. As soon as you take the fennel and leek out of the oven, transfer them to the pan with the onions and then add the rest of the stock.

Turn the heat up, bringing the soup to a simmer for 10 minutes.

Take the pan off the heat and transfer the contents to a blender. Add the cilantro and the lemon juice and blend until smooth. Check the temperature of the soup—it should be hot enough, but if not pop it back in the pan and reheat. Serve piping hot and garnish with a delicate leaf from the top of the fennel, if you like.

TASH'S TIPS
If you don't have time to roast your fennel, you can put it in raw and just increase the cooking time, so that the fennel is cooked until soft.

NUTRITIONAL NUGGET
Fennel helps to regulate hormones and provides fiber, folate, and potassium to support heart health.

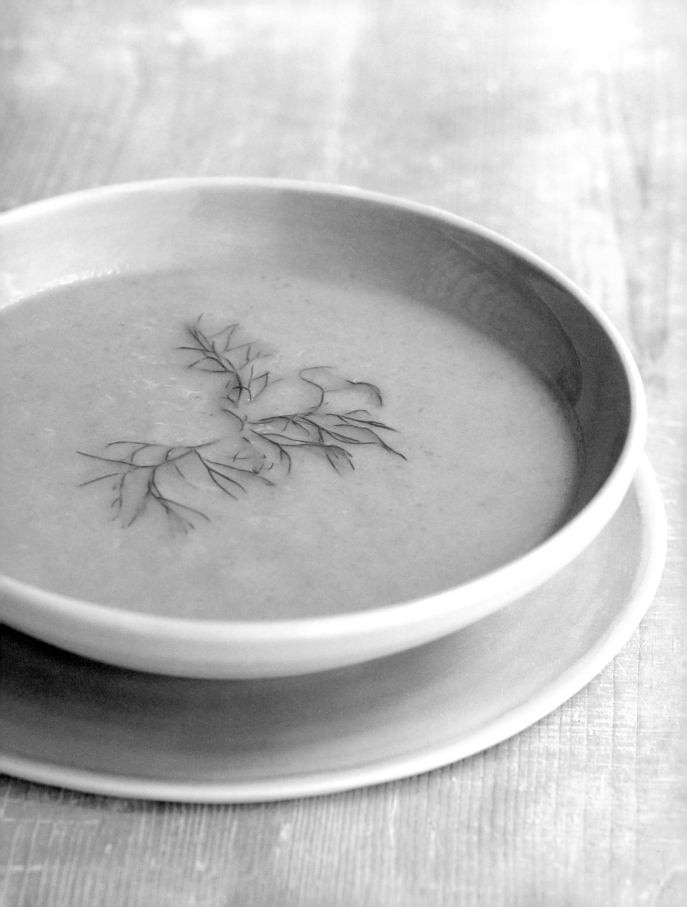

JUICES

HANGOVER NO. 2

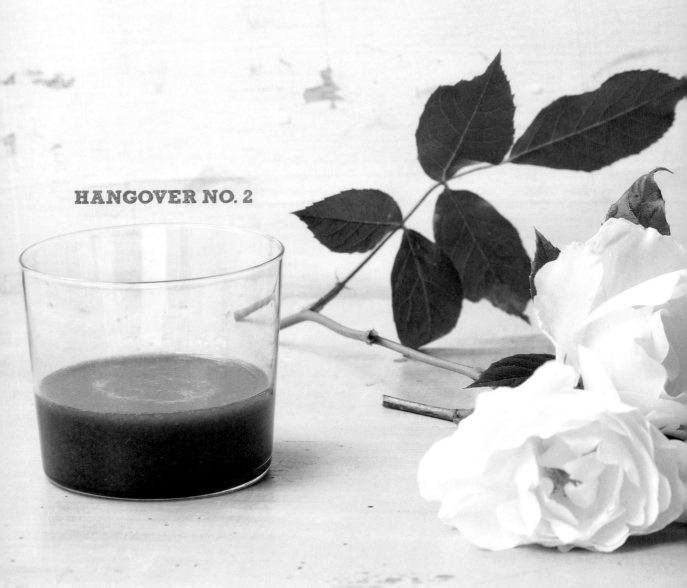

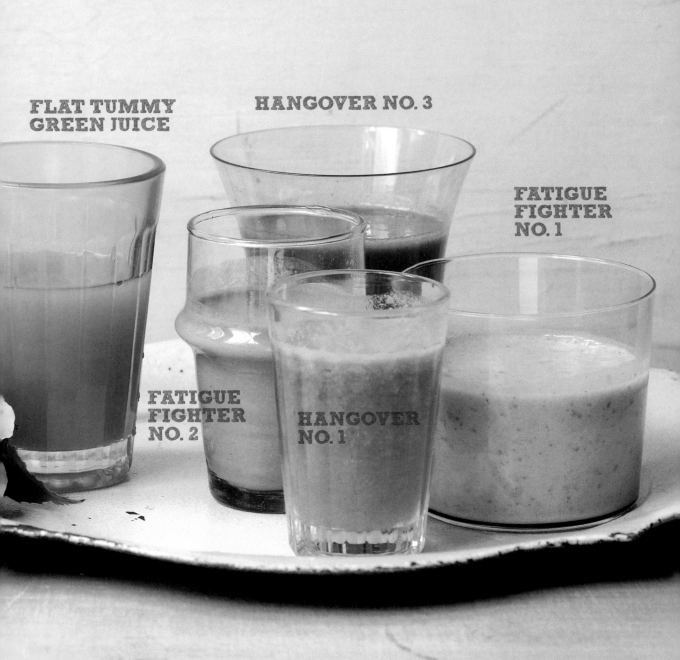

FLAT TUMMY
GREEN JUICE

HANGOVER NO. 3

FATIGUE
FIGHTER
NO. 1

FATIGUE
FIGHTER
NO. 2

HANGOVER
NO. 1

HANGOVER CURES

Hangover Cure №1

Ginger is a potent liver supporter and reduces nausea, while the coconut water rehydrates rapidly—it has the same pH as blood—helping to rebalance the sodium:potassium balance in the body. Tomatoes and lime juice supply a whack of beta-carotene and vitamin C, each of which is essential for mopping up the free radicals caused by overdrinking.

serves 1

1 tsp grated ginger root

2 medium tomatoes, roughly chopped

1½ cups coconut water

1 tsp flat-leaf parsley, chopped

juice of 1 lime

Blend all the ingredients together in a high-speed blender and pour over ice—drink immediately.

Hangover Cure №2

This cure is for the seriously hungover only. The wheatgrass or barley grass in this juice supports the liver in its detoxification process, while cucumber offers a super-alkaline base, rebalancing the body quickly. Chia is high in fiber and in essential fats to help remove the toxic waste from overindulgence.

serves 1

1 tsp wheatgrass or barley grass powder

handful of watercress, rinsed thoroughly and
   any woody stems removed

1 apple, cored and chopped

1 chia shot or 2 tsp chia seeds

½ cucumber

1 cup filtered or alkaline water

Put all the ingredients into a high-speed blender and blend until smooth, adding more water if necessary. Serve immediately for best effect.

Hangover Cure №3

Iceberg lettuce is rich in potassium and phosphorus, helping the body to redress essential electrolytes quickly. The parsley, green bell pepper, and kiwi are all great sources of vitamin C, which is used up by the body in great quantities when you have been drinking alcohol.

serves 1

½ tsp ground horseradish

½ a head of iceberg lettuce, chopped

½ green bell pepper

1 handful of flat-leaf parsley, stems removed

1 kiwi, skin removed

1 cup filtered or alkaline water

Put all the ingredients into a high-speed blender and blend until smooth, adding more water if necessary. Serve immediately for best effect.

NUTRITIONAL NUGGET
This applies to hangovers of any type! Hangovers occur as a result of extreme dehydration and it is vital to rehydrate with nutrient-laden vitamins and minerals, rather than simply water for the fastest route to rebalancing the body.

FATIGUE FIGHTERS

Fatigue Fighter №1

Almond milk is a rich source of protein, and combined with the chia seeds and oats, provides a slow-release, high energy meal-in-a-glass. The fruits add natural sweetness, without upsetting the blood sugar levels.

serves 1

1 tbsp oats

1 tsp chia seeds

1 small banana

2 dates, pits removed

1 peach or nectarine

2 drops vanilla extract

¾ cup almond milk

Blend all the ingredients together in a high-speed blender into a creamy smoothie. Drink straightaway—it really is a meal in a glass.

Fatigue Fighter №2

Avocado and cashew nuts both provide protein to boost energy for several hours. Maca powder is known for its powers of endurance, and coconut water provides slow-release energy and alkalinity.

serves 1

½ avocado

1 apple, deseeded and chopped

1 tsp maca powder

1½ cups coconut water

6–8 raw cashew nuts

Blend all the ingredients together in a high-speed blender until smooth and drink immediately, or store in an airtight container for a day in the refrigerator.

FLAT TUMMY GREEN JUICE

Fennel and celery are both excellent diuretic foods, helping the body to get rid of any excess fluid. The apple is high in pectin and fiber, which ensures that food transit time through the gut is quick, encouraging a flat tummy. In addition, probiotics help to maintain a healthy population of good digestive bacteria in the large intestine.

serves 1

1 bulb fennel

3 celery stalks, near the heart rather than outer stems

1 apple

generous 1 cup steaming water from cooking asparagus or globe artichokes (never throw away this water as it is highly alkalizing)

1 packet of probiotic powder (optional)

Juice the fennel, celery, and apple and mix together with the asparagus or artichoke water. Add the probiotic powder just before drinking, if desired. This juice lasts 6 hours if stored in the refrigerator in an airtight container.

INDEX

DIRECTORY OF SUPPLIERS

At Honestly Healthy we source everything we can locally. Here is a list of some excellent online and local suppliers. We're sure you'll soon have your own to add.

Carrying over 400 products, **Bob's Red Mill Natural Foods** has almost every kind of flour (including gluten-free options) and whole grain you can imagine
www.bobsredmill.com

The Chia Co. for their best-quality chia seed
www.thechiaco.com.au

E3Live and all other food-state supplements to add to juices and smoothies
www.e3live.com

Sold under the **Frontier Natural Products Co-op** and **Simply Organic** brands, this line of natural and organic products includes herbs, spices, and extracts
www.frontiercoop.com

Herbs, Etc. offers a large variety of herbal products
www.herbsetc.com

JaxCoco for their pure coconut water
jaxcoco.com

Navitas Naturals specializes in 100% organic superfoods that are minimally processed, gluten-free, and kosher
www.navitasnaturals.com

For their baobab, maca, spirulina, wheatgrass, and acai powdered superfoods, **Organic Burst**
www.organicburst.com

The go-to source for all things quinoa, **Quinoa Corporation** features certified organic ingredients
www.quinoa.net

For fantastic supplements, check out **Sunwarrior**
www.sunwarrior.com

Trader Joe's has many all-natural and organic products
www.traderjoes.com

You can find pretty much everything you need at **WholeFoods Market**
www.wholefoodsmarket.com

Alkaline Retreats

Contact Vicki Edgson directly if you'd like information on alkaline eating retreats.
retreats@vickiedgson.com

BIG THANK YOUS

From Tash—I want to firstly thank Jacqui and her team for believing in me a second time and having the vision to create this beautiful book. To the utterly fabulous Lisa Linder who continues to take the most stunning photos to help make this book what it is. Thanks, too, to Lawrence and Cynthia for making what we created look so gloriously beautiful and to Nikki for making sure everything made sense!

To my team at Honestly Healthy for helping to see my vision and execute my creations on the photographic shoots.

Thank you to my friends and family for being my guinea pigs over and over again, especially my trusty dinner party guests, Lucy, Bill, Wifey, Nick, Fluff, and Ike.

And to my family—they let me steal their recipes and make them Honestly Healthy! And, of course, to Vicki my partner in nutritional crime!

From Vicki—To Tash, for pushing the boat out, and having me believe that we can "have our cake and eat it too," when I was initially so resistant! To Jacqui's phenomenal team for pressing for the very best, at every level. To Lawrence, for understanding that the two parts of this book should support each other, and not be separate, and to Lisa for her jaw-droppingly beautiful photography that captures the true essence of yummy, nutritious food. And to you, the reader, for buying this book in the first place! I promise you won't be disappointed.

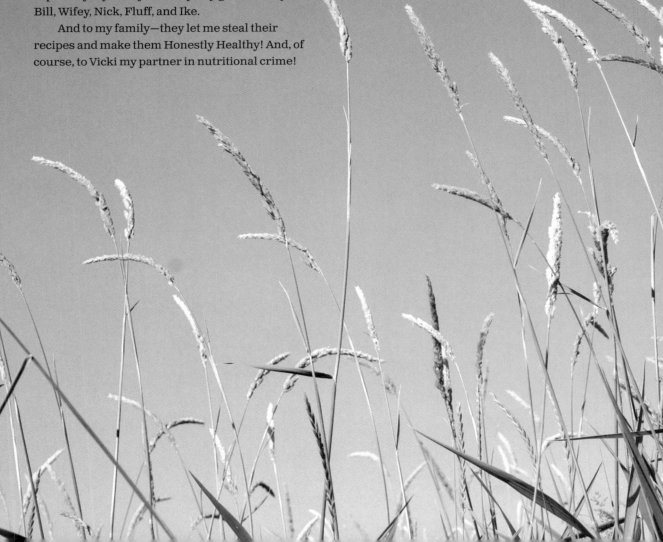

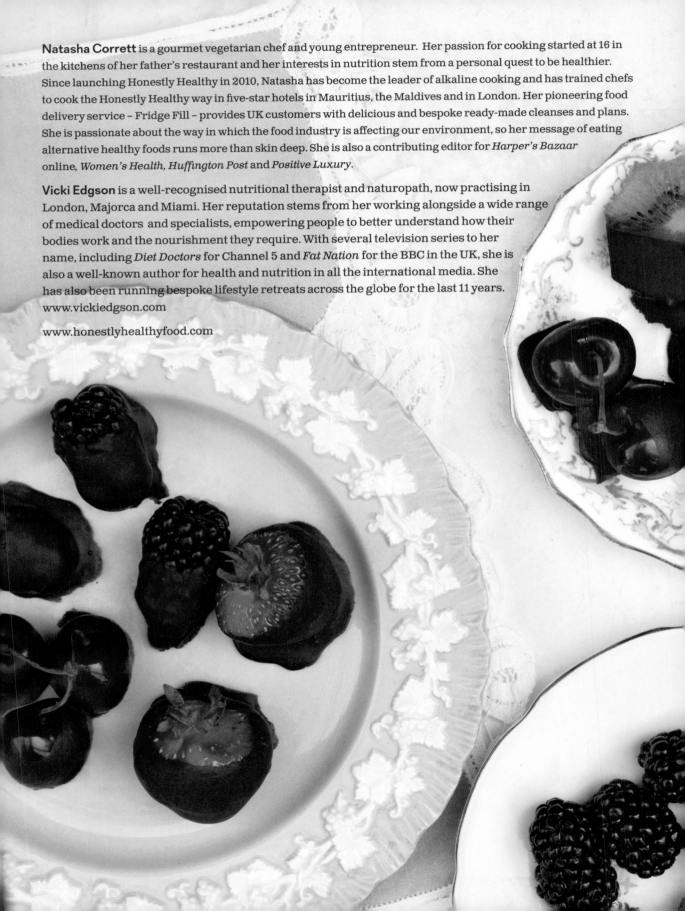

Natasha Corrett is a gourmet vegetarian chef and young entrepreneur. Her passion for cooking started at 16 in the kitchens of her father's restaurant and her interests in nutrition stem from a personal quest to be healthier. Since launching Honestly Healthy in 2010, Natasha has become the leader of alkaline cooking and has trained chefs to cook the Honestly Healthy way in five-star hotels in Mauritius, the Maldives and in London. Her pioneering food delivery service – Fridge Fill – provides UK customers with delicious and bespoke ready-made cleanses and plans. She is passionate about the way in which the food industry is affecting our environment, so her message of eating alternative healthy foods runs more than skin deep. She is also a contributing editor for *Harper's Bazaar* online, *Women's Health, Huffington Post* and *Positive Luxury*.

Vicki Edgson is a well-recognised nutritional therapist and naturopath, now practising in London, Majorca and Miami. Her reputation stems from her working alongside a wide range of medical doctors and specialists, empowering people to better understand how their bodies work and the nourishment they require. With several television series to her name, including *Diet Doctors* for Channel 5 and *Fat Nation* for the BBC in the UK, she is also a well-known author for health and nutrition in all the international media. She has also been running bespoke lifestyle retreats across the globe for the last 11 years. www.vickiedgson.com

www.honestlyhealthyfood.com